Pluripotent Stem Cells: Therapeutic Perspectives and Ethical Issues

John Libbey Eurotext
127, avenue de la République
92120 Montrouge
Tél.: 33 (0) 1 46 73 06 60
e-mail: contact@john-libbey-eurotext.fr
http://www.john-libbey-eurotext.fr

John Libbey and Company Ltd
Collier House,
163-169 Brompton Road, Knightsbridge
London SW3 1 PY, England
Tel.: 44 (0) 20 75 81 24 49

CIC Edizioni Internazionali
Corso Trieste 42
00198 Roma, Italia
Tel.: 39 06 841 26 73

© John Libbey Eurotext, 2001
ISBN: 2-7420-0369-X

All rights reserved. No part of this publication may be reproduced without written permission from the Publisher or the Centre Français du Copyright, 20, rue des Grands-Augustins, 75006 Paris.

Pluripotent Stem Cells: Therapeutic Perspectives and Ethical Issues

International Workshop
organized by
the Marcel Mérieux Foundation
21-23 June 2000

Edited by
Betty Dodet
Marissa Vicari

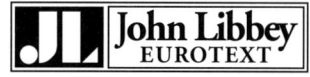

Contents

Foreword
Betty Dodet 7

Introduction
Claude Huriet 9

Implementation of complete differentiation programs by lineage precursor cell lines
Odile Kellermann, Marie Boucquey, Danièle Lamblin, Sophie Mouillet-Richard, Morgane Locker, Anne Poliard 13

Directed differentiation of dendritic cells from mouse embryonic stem cells: a novel tool for identifying targets for immunotherapy
Paul J. Fairchild, Frances A. Brook, Richard L. Gardner, Luis Graça, Victoria Strong, Yukiko Tone, Masahide Tone, Kathleen F. Nolan, Herman Waldmann .. 25

Bone marrow-derived myogenic stem cells: a therapeutic alternative for muscular dystrophy?
Giulio Cossu, Fulvio Mavilio 39

Ethical, legal and regulatory issues in the use of human embryonic stem cells in France
Claire Bonnat-Legras 45

Ethical and biological aspects concerning the use of human embryonic stem cells and the legal situation in Germany
Gisela Badura-Lotter 55

Ethical, legal and regulatory issues in the use of human embryonic stem cells in the United Kingdom
Sheila A.M. McLean 63

The moral status of the embryo and the politics of human stem cell research
Andrew W. Siegel 73

Are all cells derived from an embryo themselves embryos?
Norman Ford 81

Discussion
Marissa Vicari 89

List of contributors 95

Pluripotent Stem Cells: Therapeutic Perspectives and Ethical Issues
B. Dodet, M. Vicari, eds.
© John Libbey Eurotext, Paris, 2001

Foreword

In 1987, under the guidance of its president Dr Charles Mérieux, the Mérieux Foundation considered the question of the statute of the human embryo. Dr Louis Valette organised at Lyon, with the Catholic University, an interdisciplinary discussion on ethical questions raised by new techniques in the field of medically assisted reproduction.

At the moment when, in France, the bioethics laws have come up for review, questions regarding the statute of the embryo return to the heart of scientific debates. Breakthroughs in the field of embryonic stem cell biology offer a glimpse of the considerable therapeutic possibilities. Research Institutes and Governments, hailed by these new therapeutic perspectives, are attempting to put in place modes of regulating this research that both respond to citizen's aspirations and conform to ethical norms.

This work is comprised of the presentations and debates that took place during a colloquium on pluripotent stem cells held at the Mérieux Foundation Conference Centre, which united for a period of three days researchers, ethicists, philosophers, representatives of different faiths, lawyers, politicians, academics and professionals of biotechnology industry. Here are assembled certain texts from presentations on cellular biology research: the establishment and differentiation of embryonic stem cell lines (Odile Kellermann, Paul Fairchild *et al.*) and adult stem cells (Giulio Cossu and Fulvio Mavilio). The presentations concerning the ethical and legal aspects of the utilisation of stem cells, with the issues presented by Senator Huriet, address the legal and regulatory situations regarding the use of stem cells in France (Claire Bonnat), Germany (Gisela Badura-Lotter), the United Kingdom (Sheila McLean) and the United States (Andrew Siegel). Certain manuscripts had to be revised during the compilation of this work, to integrate new information and new stands and decisions taken by the various governments. The question of the statute of embryonic stem cells – should they be considered as embryos? – is framed by Reverend Norman Ford. Themes that animated the discussion of this session are taken up in the chapter by Marissa Vicari.

We would like to thank here all those who contributed to the realisation of this event, particularly Senator Huriet who accepted to chair the session consecrated to ethics and to prepare the introduction. We would like to express our sincere appreciation for his participation.

Betty Dodet
Scientific Director
Mérieux Foundation

Pluripotent Stem Cells: Therapeutic Perspectives and Ethical Issues
B. Dodet, M. Vicari, eds.
© John Libbey Eurotext, Paris, 2001

Introduction

Claude Huriet
Senator of Meurthe-et-Moselle, France
Parliamentary Office for Evaluation of Scientific and Technological Options, Paris, France

A top-level international seminar consecrated to pluripotent stem cells – that is, ES cells – provides an opportunity for scientists of all backgrounds to review and exchange information on the current state of their research; it is also an exceptional occasion for reflecting on the specific ethical problems of the "bio-sciences" raised by the eventual utilisation of the human embryo for the realisation of the many therapeutic aims that have been recently postulated.

Recently... it was in fact in November 1998 that the prolonged culture of human embryonic and germinal stem cells, and their therapeutic perspectives, appeared. In little more than two years, much research has been done, allowing us to foresee the expanse of domains in which embryonic stem cells may bring a revolution in the prognostic of a certain number of currently incurable afflictions, for example, neurodegenerative diseases or cardiac disease.

In the past few months, while we have barely begun to contemplate the possibilities of controlled cell differentiation, we have seen that stem cells derived from bone marrow may, under certain conditions, differentiate into neurons, myocardial and hepatic cells, thus marking a new and promising step.

The research continues, our understanding grows, and progress, in this field as in others, accelerates.

This acceleration of progress demands a certain intellectual exaltation, to nourish the illusion of the omnipotence of mankind, as the master of life and of its own destiny.

Scientists in the life sciences may get a feeling of unlimited power if they don't pause from time to time and reflect on life, its origin, the effects of their work, and the values upon which their work is based. Ethical reflection has become inescapable and necessary; all researchers are confronted, whether they admit it or not, by questions to which they cannot provide "the" best answer, and it is essential that they leave their solitude behind from time to time to discover what others are thinking!

The Mérieux Foundation's seminar on pluripotent stem cells provided the opportunity to do exactly that, evincing a common perception of the problem, with identical questions, but – not surprisingly – with responses to difficult questions which were often quite different.

According to the commonly accepted definition, ES cells, derived from the internal cell mass of the blastocyst, are "pluripotent" because they cannot produce an embryo, at least in the absence of trophoblast cells.

More delicate is the definition of the embryo, such that Reverend Norman Ford proposed the following definition: *"an isolated living cell or multicellular organism, which innately possesses the real capacity to realise its species specific development, that is to say its human development, when in an appropriate environment"*. Norman Ford insists upon the essential philosophical distinction between the cells *which develop to become* a human embryo and an embryo which, at the moment of fertilisation, *becomes* an embryo derived from an ovule and a spermatazoid.

Cited by Gisella Badura-Lotter, the German embryo protection law defines the embryo as: *"the fertilised human ovule, capable of development, derived from the fusion of germ cells, as well as any totipotent cell derived from an embryo, capable of dividing and developing into an individual under favourable conditions"*.

The recurring dilemma raised by the six speakers comprising the "ethics session" of the seminar revealed the origin of the analyses concerning the current possibilities and perspectives of the utilisation of ES cells and the aims of research.

The current possibilities and perspectives opened by ES cells concern research and the development of new treatments: identification of the mechanisms which govern cellular differentiation with the aim of directing the differentiation of pluripotent stem cells in order to obtain differentiated cell lines (A.W. Siegel), including neurons and muscle and blood cells or other "cell therapies" with many possible applications.

The utilisation of stem cells derived from animals may concern the trials and toxicological studies of new medicines and their toxic side-effects on embryos. Regarding the aims of research, Sheila A.M. McLean, citing the Nuffield Committee, underlines that *"research on the development of new treatments is not qualitatively different from research on fertility treatment. Neither case benefits the embryo used in research, but both cases may benefit others in the future"*. It is upon such an argument, which is difficult to contest, that the ethical debate on the utilisation of the human embryo is founded.

As well as a common perception of the problem, the speakers shared the same ethical questions. In fact, if the responses currently given regarding the utilisation of human embryos differ, from a distance, the dilemma is the following:

– the human embryo merits respect and it is inadmissible to treat it as an object by denying it the possibility of implantation after its creation;

– an embryo has been created with the goal of being implanted into a uterus. If it is not implanted, it has no future. Under these conditions, the sampling and culturing of cells from this embryo does not signal a lack of respect (Nuffield Report).

Another question, formulated by Norman Ford, regards cells derived from the embryo: are they all, themselves, embryos? If we refer to the definitions proposed above, the response could only be negative. A mass of ES cells – pluripotent and not totipotent

– without trophoblast cells, cannot become an embryo capable of the specific development of the human species.

Contrary to the disposition of the 1990 *English Human Fertilisation and Embryology Act* (HFE), which authorises research on embryos under 14 days old, a delay which to many seems arbitrary, these data collected on embryos demonstrate that the "ethical debate" is related not only to the cells as such, but to their derivation from embryos, the conditions of their sampling and the consequences of this derivation for the embryo.

Considering an evaluation of the same problem and identical formations of the ethical questions, one can only be surprised by the diversity of responses. Apparently, the origin of this diversity stems from different cultural, philosophical or spiritual references. All the same, it is situated outside of the sphere of purely rational analysis, such that the scientific debate is confronted with values which designate limits.

In Great Britain, the HFE permits the creation of embryos for research with certain fixed and limited objectives, as well as research on donated embryos. On the other hand, the German Embryo Protection Act prohibits all *in vitro* experimentation on the human embryo not in the interest of the embryo concerned, thus prohibiting the production of cultured ES cells. In the United States (A.W. Siegel), a controversy has developed concerning the moral and political aspects of ES cell research. The existing legislation is quite varied. Research on the human embryo and on human embryonic cell lines is not regulated if financed by private funds ; however, it is prohibited or limited in ten states. No federal funding may be allocated to the creation of human embryos for research or for research involving the destruction of human embryos. The question of whether ES cells *"which are not themselves embryos"* are covered by the law, was recently posed. The most recent text to date (August 20, 2000) prohibits public financing of the *derivation* of human embryonic stem cells, but authorises the *utilisation* of these cells in research! And the debate, between members of Congress proposing a law prohibiting all federal funding of research with human ES cells and those demanding that public funds be available for the derivation as well as the use of these cells, is not yet closed.

In France, the 1994 "bioethics" laws contain the following dispositions: an embryo cannot be created for commercial or industrial ends; it may not be created *in vitro* for study, research or experimentation. All experimentation on the embryo is prohibited. In exceptional cases, studies which do not harm the embryo may be performed. The review of the 1994 law, which was to occur five years after its promulgation, is on hold, and we cannot yet evaluate whatever alterations might be made. The Conseil d'Etat, in a report made public in November 1999, sought *"a fair balance between respect for life from its beginning and the right of those who suffer to see society undertake the most efficient research possible, in the fight against their illnesses"* (Claire Bonnat). It is difficult to say whether such an equilibrium may be obtained.

We can see that the responses based on current laws differ fundamentally from one country to another and that the result may carry formidable consequences. In fact, where the perspectives of the therapeutic utilisation of stem cells are most assured, the pressure is the strongest to lift bans where they exist. A.W. Siegel noted that establishing in the law a distinction between the derivation, which implies the destruction of the embryo, and the utilisation of stem cells obtained by a third party is not ethically satisfactory: *"the scientists who use stem cells obtained by a third party may also be considered as morally complicit to the destruction of the embryos. Ethically speaking, it's a little as if one were to engage a hit man."* G. Badura-Lotter raised a hypothesis according to which, in Germany, the import of ES cells from other countries where the utilisation of embryos in research is allowed, may be authorised in accordance with a disposition of the penal code, *lex loci*, which ties culpability to the state in which the crime was committed, in the case of pluripotent (and not totipotent) stem cells.

It could be said that the exchanges fostered by the Merieux Foundation's seminar were "passionate," in the sense that passion was not absent from the debates! The therapeutic perspectives opened by the utilisation of pluripotent stem cells are very real, even if the time scale is at present unknown. It is, however, today that scientists and society are confronted by a dramatic choice between respect for the human person, albeit it potential, according to the formulation of the French National Consultative Ethics Committee, and the hopes of numerous ill people of being cured.

Among the possibilities recently discussed, that of inducing differentiation of human adult stem cells to yield different types of cells for therapy was recalled several times. It is evident that they provide a solution which bypasses the current issues. While they certainly don't constitute a sort of convenient alibi for, they are already supported by such solid experimental evidence that we would be wrong not to consider their investigation.

Pluripotent Stem Cells: Therapeutic Perspectives and Ethical Issues
B. Dodet, M. Vicari, eds.
© John Libbey Eurotext, Paris, 2001

Implementation of complete differentiation programs by lineage precursor cell lines

Odile Kellermann[1], Marie Boucquey[2], Danièle Lamblin[1], Sophie Mouillet-Richard[1], Morgane Locker[1], Anne Poliard[1]

[1] Unité de Génétique Somatique, Institut Pasteur, Paris, France
[2] Ludwig Institute for Cancer Research, Brussels Branch, and Cellular Genetics Unit, Université Catholique de Louvain, Bruxelles, Belgique

Summary – Our studies focus on the mechanisms of commitment and differentiation of stem cell lines of neuroectodermal, mesodermal or endodermal origin. We have developed an immortalization strategy based upon the introduction of a recombinant adenovirus-SV40 plasmid (PK4) into multipotential cells and have isolated new *in vitro* differentiation models. The immortalized clones display the properties of stem cells characterized by (i) a homogenous, stable and undifferentiated phenotype (self-renewal), (ii) the expression of genes involved in the differentiation of early embryonic cells after gastrulation and (iii) the capacity to undergo complete differentiation along alternative pathways of the same lineage.

The murine F9-derived 1C11 clone exhibits a stable epithelial morphology, expresses nestin, an early neuroectodermal marker, and genes involved in neuroectodermal cell fate. Upon appropriate induction, 100% of 1C11 precursor cells develop neurite extensions and acquire neuronal markers (N-CAM, synaptophysin, $\gamma\gamma$-enolase, and neurofilament) as well as the general functions of either serotoninergic or noradrenergic neurons. The two programs are mutually exclusive. The time-dependent onset of neurotransmitter-associated functions proper to either program is similar to *in vivo* observations. Along each pathway, the selective induction of serotoninergic or adrenergic receptors is an essential part of the differentiation program, since they promote autoregulation of the corresponding phenotype.

This neuronal cell line constitutes a tool for characterizing the serotonin transporter (target of antidepressant) within an integrated serotoninergic context and identifying the intracellular targets and the crosstalks between the signalling pathways of the 5-HT$_{1B/1D}$, 5-HT$_{2B}$ and 5-HT$_{2A}$ receptors. *In vivo*, the concentration of serotonin (5-hydroxytryptamine, 5-HT) is highly regulated, and deregulation induces major neuropsychiatric and cardiovascular disorders. In this context, it is of interest to understand how a clonal serotoninergic cell line such as 1C11 regulates through its 5-HT receptors, the metabolism, storage and transport of 5-HT as well as the expression of neuronal functions, depending on the external 5-HT concentration. Similarly, the 1C11 cell line may help gain insight into the regulation of noradrenergic differentiation by α_{1D} adrenoreceptors.

The tripotential mesodermal C1 clone has the capacity to follow all the steps leading to osteogenic, chondrogenic or adipogenic terminal differentiation depending on the nature of the inducers. Again, the frequency of differentiation is over 80% and the three pathways are mutually exclusive. The C1 clone constitutes an *in vitro* model to study the mechanisms governing mesodermal cell fate decision. It also allows the identification of the paracrine and autocrine effectors underlying chondrogenesis from the stem cell state to the hypertrophic cartilage state when mature cells prepare for endochondral bone formation.

Studying the relative part of genetic and epigenetic regulation in the control of specialized cellular functions *in vivo* or in heterogenous primary cultures remains an arduous task. Inducible somatic stem cell lines are aimed at analyzing how the differentiation program of a precursor cell is ruled (i) by its intrinsic genetic program, *i.e.* the memory originating from its ancestors along a lineage, and (ii) by the environmental signals activating intracellular signalling pathways. Lineage precursor cell lines also pave the way towards the identification of stem cell specific markers which would facilitate their *in vivo* localization and *in vitro* selection for somatic cell therapy.

An immortalization strategy designed to establish lineage precursor cell lines from multipotent cells

Differentiation may be defined as the set of processes that allow a cell to acquire, maintain and modulate its specialized functions. *In vivo*, differentiated cells are programmed to undergo cell death. Stem cells only are immortal, *i.e.* have the capacity both to self-renew and to give rise, upon induction, to a progeny that may irreversibly go through all the steps of a differentiation program up to its terminal stages. Still, in the adult, little is known about the very sparse stem cells which take part in tissue renewal and repair. In the embryo, multipotential cells give rise to stem cells during gastrulation. Our approach is based upon multipotential cell lines as a source for isolating lineage stem cells and for developing new *in vitro* differentiation models. Teratocarcinoma-derived EC or ES multipotential cells have the capacity to mimick *in vitro* the early differentiation steps of the embryonic inner cell mass along the embryonic and extraembryonic lineages. However, the cells stop dividing as they loose their multipotentiality and this precludes the cloning and selection of pure committed progenitor cell lines among the heterogenous EC- or ES-derived cultures. Moreover, the inducers driving unidirectional differentiation of multipotential cells along a specific lineage are yet to be identified. The challenge was thus to introduce oncogenes which would permit immortalization of lineage precursor cell lines without preventing their potential of differentiation.

Our immortalization strategy *(figure 1)* was designed through the construction of the PK4 plasmid in which SV40 oncogenes are under the control of the type 5 adenovirus E1A promoter [1]. Adenovirus is among the few viruses to be expressed in the early developmental stages of mouse embryogenesis [2]. Embryonal carcinoma multipotential cells were transfected with PK4 and then induced to differentiate. The E1A promoter allows the expression of SV40 oncogenes during the early stages of multipotential cell differentiation, at the very beginning of commitment. An immortalized population of immature and differentiated cells of neuroectodermal, mesodermal or endodermal origin was obtained [3-6].

Immature cells likely corresponding to potential lineage precursor stem cells were cloned and selected on the basis of the following criteria: (i) loss of expression of multipotential cell markers, *i.e.* irreversible loss of cell multipotentiality; (ii) expression of the SV40 T antigen and immortalization; (iii) stable immature phenotype; (iv) reproductibility of differentiation towards a unique lineage, either *in vitro* or *in vivo* in tumours, after injection in nude or irradiated mice.

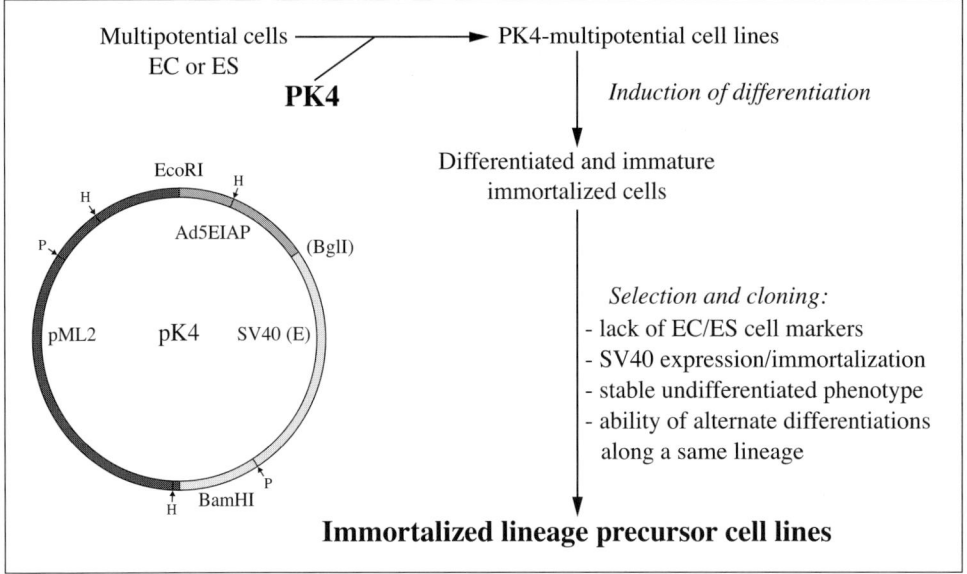

Figure 1. Immortalization strategy through an adenovirus-SV40 (pK4) hybrid plasmid.

Among the many immortalized cell lines of neuroectodermal, endodermal and mesodermal origin, we favoured the characterization of the 1C11 and C1 stem cells which constitute novel models to study neuronal or mesodermal differentiation. Such multipotential cell-derived precursors have never been isolated before from primary cultures nor from transgenic mice or transgenic embryos nor even from tumours.

Studying these cell lines led us first to identify the inducers specific for each program, then to describe the kinetics of acquisition of differentiation markers. This was enabled by the synchrony and the high frequency of phenotypic conversion up to terminal differentiation. Thus, although immortalized, these progenitor clones retain the capacity to differentiate towards alternative pathways along a lineage depending on the nature of the inducing agent(s). Lineage precursor cell lines allow to investigate into differentiation mechanisms which cannot be easily unraveled *in vivo* or on heterogenous cell cultures. We are pursuing their characterization and evaluating the role of a series of effectors (transcription factors, hormones, neuromediators, growth factors, drugs, cellular interactions...) on the onset and integration of the specialized cell functions. This should favour an analysis of the cellular response to a paracrine or autocrine signal in relation to the differentiation state of the cell and the identification of the intracellular targets that are newly synthetized or modified (phosphorylation/dephosphorylation, transcriptional and/or post-transcriptional controls...) following this signal.

The isolation of lineage precursor cell lines aims at understanding (i) how a somatic stem cell phenotype is controlled and what its specific markers are; hallmark(s) characteristic of precursor cells should favour the *in vivo* identification of stem cells for the development of gene therapy; (ii) how specialized genetic programs are turned on from this immature "committed" state, *i.e.* what are the mechanisms that recruit the stem cell, control its choice of fate and ensure the implementation of the differentiated phenotype in a self-autonomous manner; (iii) how an immature or a terminally differentiated cell regulates its metabolism and functions in response to the signals it receives.

A neuroectodermal cell line inducible towards a serotoninergic or a noradrenergic program

The 1C11 cell line results from the direct *in vitro* induction of F9-PK4 multipotential cells by retinoic acid and dbcAMP [1, 4]. The 1C11 clone has lost multipotentiality, and, considering its origin, most likely corresponds to a very early progenitor. As a genuine stem cell, the 1C11 clone exhibits unlimited "self-renewal" capacity maintaining an epithelial and immature phenotype under long-term standard culture conditions. It does not express any neuronal functions such as N-CAM, neurofilaments and neurotransmitter biosynthetic enzymes and never spontaneously generates a differentiated progeny, even in 10% serum-supplemented medium. The homogenous expression of L-CAM and nestin, a neuroepithelial marker, further characterizes 1C11 as an immature neuroectodermal precursor [6]. The 1C11 clone behaves as a bipotential neuronal stem cell capable of differentiating into fully functional serotoninergic or noradrenergic neuronal-like cells *(figure 2)*.

Therefore, despite the lack of a proper embryonal environment, the conversion of F9 multipotential cells into 1C11 committed cells seems to correspond to an irreversible lineage restriction towards the neural fate. Hallmarks specific of neuroepithelial progenitors are not yet available and the cellular identity and the developmental stage of 1C11 cannot yet be established with certainty. Screening for genes differentially expressed in 1C11 and in its parental cell line (Marie Boucquey, current work) may further facilitate the identification of new cell markers characteristic of immature neuroectodermal progenitors.

Cell fate decision taken by neural ectoderm cells is influenced by a variety of signals, either endogenous, such as developmentally expressed bioamines [7] and neurotrophins, or exogenous, originating from the somites and the notochord [8]. Among the complex network of pathways that dictates the developmental choice of neural progenitors, the Notch signaling pathway is of critical importance. The combined expression in 1C11 cells of transcripts encoding Notch-1 to 3 and the corresponding ligands, Delta and Jagged, together with the homogenous immunostaining of the cells nuclei [6] with Notch-1 antibodies suggests that Notch-ligand interactions take part in determining the fate of 1C11 cells. Furthermore, the 1C11 precursor expresses transcripts encoding Krox-20, a protein of the developing hindbrain [9], as well as low levels of mRNAs corresponding to MASH-1, the mammalian homologue of the Drosophila Achaete-scute proneural genes [10]. The expression of MASH-1 mRNAs in 1C11 cells is consistent with the overlapping expression of MASH-1 and Notch-1 observed during early mouse central nervous system development [10]. All these genes play important – albeit not entirely understood – roles in early neurogenesis and patterning of the nervous system. Their co-expression with nestin in 1C11 cells, indicates that the 1C11 clone may correspond to a neuroepithelial stem cell. That serotoninergic and catecholaminergic cells

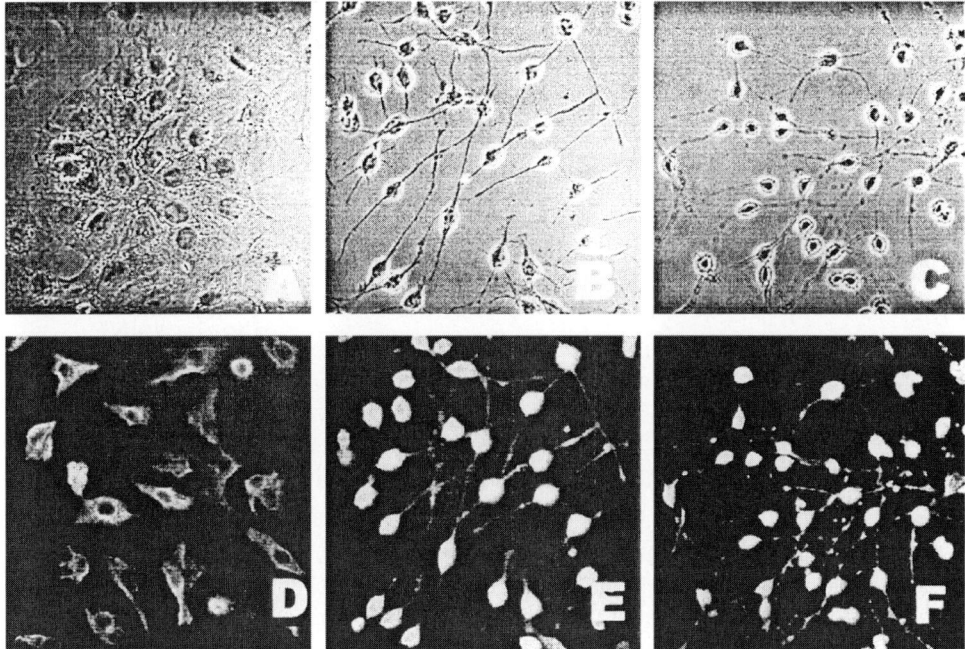

Figure 2. Immunocytochemical characterization of the 1C11 neuroepithelial precursor cell and its resulting 1C11*/5HT serotoninergic and 1C11**/NE catecholaminergic progeny.
(A) Phase contrast pictures of the 1C11 neuroepithelial precursor cell and its resulting (B) 1C11*/5HT serotoninergic or (C) 1C11**/NE catecholaminergic progeny. Homogenous staining of (D) 1C11 precursor cells with antibodies against nestin; (E) 1C11*/5HT serotoninergic cells at day 4 with antibodies against 5-HT and (F) 1C11**/NE catecholaminergic cells at day 4 with antibodies against NE.

may share a common precursor in the course of embryonic development has never been clearly established. However, very recent observations [11] suggest that monoaminergic neurons indeed arise from a common neural progenitor.

The differentiation steps [6] of the 1C11 precursor cell line are summarized in *figure 3*.

– 1C11 cells treated for 4 days with inducers (dbcAMP, CCA) differentiate into 1C11$^{*/5\text{-HT}}$ cells [4]. These 1C11$^{*/5\text{-HT}}$ cells express a complete serotoninergic phenotype. They synthesize, catabolize, store, recapture serotonin, and express a defined set of serotoninergic receptors (5-HT$_{2A, \, 2B, \, 1B/1D}$) [12].

– 1C11 cells treated for 12 days with dbcAMP and DMSO convert into 1C11$^{**/NE}$ cells [6]. 1C11$^{**/NE}$ cells express a complete noradrenergic phenotype. They synthesize, catabolize and store norepinephrine (NA) as soon as day 4 of differentiation; they acquire a functional NA transporter at day 12. An α_{1D} adrenoreceptor is selectively induced at day 8 of this differentiation program.

The switch between the two programs is complete; differentiations are synchronous and concern nearly 100% of cells *(figure 2)*. 1C11$^{*/5\text{-HT}}$ and 1C11$^{**/NE}$ cells coexpress neuronal markers [6] such as neurofilament, N-CAM, $\gamma\gamma$-enolase and synaptophysin.

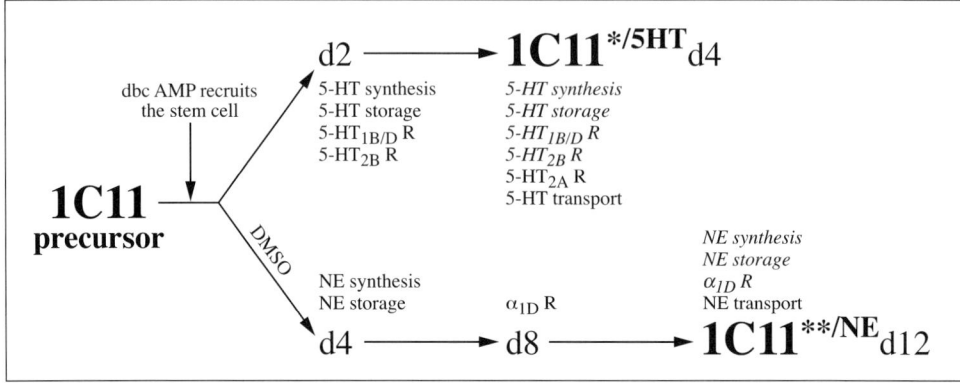

Figure 3. The different steps of 1C11 stem cell differentiation.

This differentiation model thus has three very homogenous states: the 1C11 stem cell state, the 1C11$^{*/5\text{-}HT}$ serotoninergic state, the 1C11$^{**/NE}$ catecholaminergic state.

The kinetics of both differentiations are similar to those observed *in vivo*. The 1C11$^{*/5\text{-}HT}$ cell's serotoninergic phenotype reaches completion within 4 days; similarly, in the rat, the ontogeny of central serotoninergic neurons, originating in the raphe nuclei, has been shown to occur within a definite period of 4 days, from embryonic day 11 (ED11) to ED15. As observed for 1C11$^{*/5\text{-}HT}$ cells *(figure 3)*, neurotransmitter synthesis becomes measurable 2 days (at ED13) prior to the onset of monoamine transporters (ED15) [13]. Several features of 1C11$^{**/NE}$ differentiation are also reminiscent of the *in vivo* situation. During the program, as *in vivo* [14], the synthesis of catecholamines (TH activity) occurs prior to NE uptake. 1C11$^{**/NE}$ cells have more robust dendritic trees but shorter processes than 1C11$^{*/5\text{-}HT}$ cells *(figure 2)*, as the noradrenalin-containing neurons of the brainstem.

The serotoninergic and adrenergic receptors specifically induced along each pathway autoregulate the implementation of the respective phenotype. Three functional 5-HT receptors are sequentially induced during the serotoninergic differentiation of the 1C11 clone. 5-HT$_{2B}$ and 5-HT$_{1B/D}$ receptors are detectable at day 2 of differentiation. At day 4, a third 5-HT receptor, 5-HT$_{2A}$, becomes expressed. The functional presence of any other 5-HT receptor subtype or dopaminergic, muscarinic, glutamate, GABAergic... binding sites has been excluded [6, 12].

Under 5-HT starvation in the culture medium, the time sequence of serotoninergic differentiation remained unchanged. At day 4, however, 5-HT cellular content ($\times 2.8$), 5-HT synthesis *via* TPH activity ($\times 9.3$) and the apparent Vmax of 5-HT transport ($\times 7.7$) were higher than the values obtained with 1C11$^{*/5\text{-}HT}$ cells grown in 10% serum supplemented medium [6]. Thus 5-HT synthesized by 1C11$^{*/5\text{-}HT}$ cells exerts a negative feedback on all the serotoninergic functions *via* receptors. The 5-HT receptors regulate the entire of process metabolism and transport and the transporter which captures more or less external 5-HT acts on receptor functions.

Deciphering the mechanisms that coordinate cellular functions first requires an accurate knowledge of the receptors transduction pathways. Our priority has been to characterize the 5-HT$_{2B}$ receptor which is a new receptor expressed in the heart and the neural tube right after gastrulation of the embryo [15] and in the heart, cardiovasculature, intestine, kidney and brain of the adult. The *in vivo* signalling pathways mediating the physiological functions of 5-HT$_{2B}$ receptors remains largely unknown [16]. Nevertheless, using the 1C11 model system, 4 transduction pathways have been characterized: 5-HT$_{2B}$ receptors are coupled with the IP$_3$ [17] ras [18] signalling pathways, they can also trigger NO formation [19] and PLA2-mediated arachidonic acid (AA) release [20]. At day 2 of differentiation of 1C11$^{*/5\text{-}HT}$ cells, the activation of 5-HT$_{2B}$ receptors inhibits 5-HT$_{1B/D}$ receptor function through the PLA2/AA pathway [20]. At day 4, this inhibitory effect can be antagonized by the stimulation of 5-HT$_{2A}$ receptors. Additional signal transduction and crosstalk studies will likely allow for identification of the intracellular targets of these receptors and thereby unravel some of the molecular events leading to the coordination of serotoninergic functions.

Similarly, 1C11$^{**/NE}$ cells selectively acquire a functional adrenoceptor of the α_{1D} subtype from day 8 of noradrenergic differentiation. While not regulating the catecholaminergic metabolism, this receptor is involved in the completion of the phenotype because its blockade at day 8 impairs NE transport at day 12 [6].

The bioaminergic receptors thus act as autoreceptors taking a critical part in the achievement and epigenetic regulation of the otherwise intrinsic genetic program. *In vivo*, deregulations of the functionality of bioaminergic receptors or transporters are associated with major neuropsychiatric or cardiovascular disorders. Studies of neuromediator-associated functions on an inducible neuronal cell line expressing a definite set of receptors such as 1C11 may also have therapeutic implications.

The C1 tripotential mesodermal cell line:
an *in vitro* model to study osteogenic, chondrogenic and adipogenic differentiation from stem cell recruitment to terminal differentiation

Osteoblasts, chondroblasts and adipoblasts are believed to originate from common embryonic progenitors derived from mesodermal (somites, limb buds) and mesectodermal (neural crest) embryonic lineages. The initial steps of bone formation involve conversion of mesodermal cells into osteoblasts either directly (intramembranous ossification) or *via* intermediate stages, with cartilage matrix being progressively replaced by bone (endochondral ossification). In the adult, renewal or maintenance of bone, cartilage and fat as well as bone repair also depends on mesodermal stem cells located in the bone marrow stroma [21] and the adjacent periosteum, endosteum or perichondrium [22].

Differentiation of mesodermal stem cells up to the endstage of either osteogenesis or chondrogenesis depends on both intrinsic genetic programs and environmental signals (cell-cell or cell-matrix interactions, vitamins, cytokines). The characterization of the respective contributing factors from stem cell recruitment to tissue maintenance and repair is of utmost importance in conjunctive tissue biology and may be undertaken with *in vitro* models. We established a clone, C1, after introduction of the plasmid PK4 into the EC-1003 cell line [5]. Upon injection of multipotential 1003-PK4 EC cells into syngeneic mice, teratocarcinoma were obtained. In cultures derived from the tumors, areas containing mesodermal derivatives closely associated with immature cells were selected with the idea that the immature cells might correspond to mesodermal progenitors. The C1 cell line was cloned from an island of cells resembling the somitic mesoderm enriched in cartilage, bone, muscle and adipocyte-like cells. The C1 clone has the properties of a tripotential mesodermal precursor [23] and corresponds to an earlier step of commitment in the mesodermal lineage compared to bone or cartilage primary cultures or immortalized osteoblast or chondrocyte cell lines [21-24 and references therein].

As genuine progenitor cells, C1 cells maintain a stable and undifferentiated phenotype and can be converted at high frequency into either osteoblasts, chondrocytes or adipocytes in response to extracellular signals *(figure 4)*. Cell-cell interactions are required prior to any of these differentiation programs. These contacts turn on the expression of the early genes of all three programs and render the cells competent to be recruited. C1 cells do not differentiate spontaneously even in 10% serum supplemented medium. Beyond this stage, cells need instructive signal(s) to enter a particular differentiation pathway and to reach endstages through specific temporal regulation of gene expression. For osteogenic or chondrogenic differentiation, C1 cells must form nodules mimicking the *in vivo* cell condensation necessary for skeleton development. Our current view of the C1 model (illustrated in *figure 5*) includes the following points:

– In response to ascorbic acid (AA) and β-glycerophosphate (βGP), within 4 days close to 100% of the nodules secrete a type I collagen (col) ECM which rapidly mineralizes [5, 24, 25]. As in normal bone, calcified foci are composed of hydroxyapatite cristals on type 1 col fibers.

– Upon chronic exposure to dexamethasone (DEX) (10^{-6} M), within 4 weeks 80% of the nodules develop foci of chondrocyte-like cells having the capacity to build up an ECM mainly composed of type II col and aggrecan. Thereafter, C1 mature chondrocytes become hypertrophic and elaborate a type X col matrix typical of the terminal stages of chondrogenesis in the growth plate of long bones [23, 24].

– Finally, if cultured in monolayers, C1 confluent cells convert into functional adipocytes under the synergistic effect of DEX (10^{-7} M) and insulin (10^{-6} M) [23].

The C1 clone illustrates the power of epigenetic signals in directing the fate of pluripotent mesoblastic cell lines. Once recruited by the inducers, C1 cells adopt a defined identity with clear switch between phenotypes. Each program follows a reproducible schedule that can be divided into distinct lineage-specific stages based on changes in biochemical properties, collagen expression and matrix deposition. These changes have characteristic properties close to those documented *in vivo* [24].

Serum-free conditions (previously 1% serum) for chondrogenic differentiation have been recently set up. The mesodermal progenitor is capable of completing, *in vitro*, the chondrogenic program up to its terminal stage in the sole presence of Dex. Dex seems to be absolutely required for the recruitment of C1 chondrogenesis, but can be suppressed from the mature chondrocyte stage. Thereafter, thyroid hormone appears to be a very efficient effector in triggering phenotypic conversion towards hypertrophy. This demonstrates that a clonal mesoblastic cell line, once recruited, has the intrinsic potential to recapitulate *in vitro*, at high frequency and in a nearly synchronous manner, all steps of chondrogenesis as observed in the growth plate.

Despite the lack of a proper embryonal environment, C1 precursor cells express in a lineage- and temporal-dependent way a series of genes (BMPs, BMP-receptor, PTH,

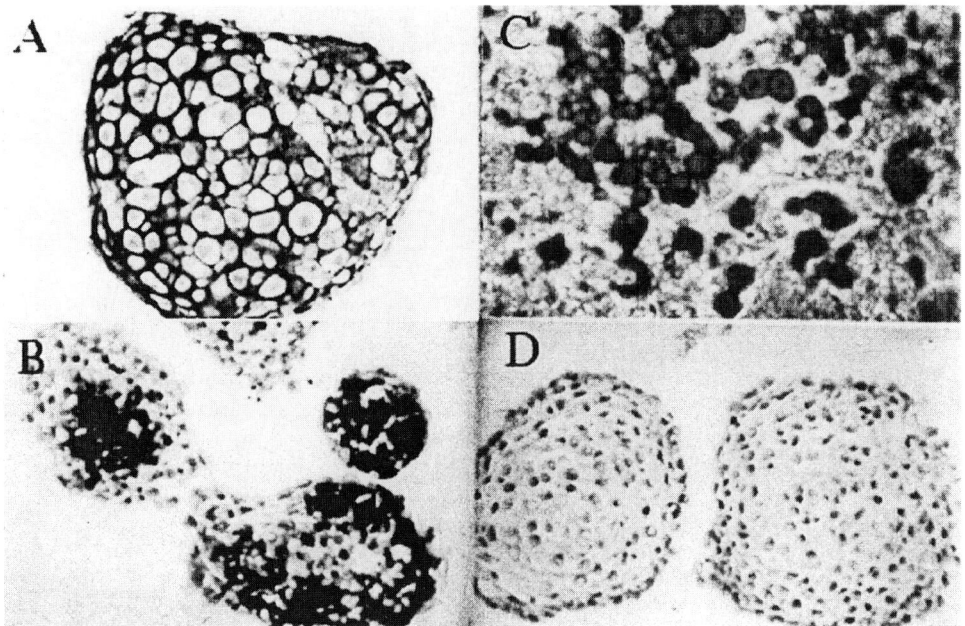

Figure 4. Phenotypic conversion of C1 cells into osteocyte-, chondrocyte-, and adipocyte-like cells.
(A) DEX-treated nodules at 40 days of culture showing mature chondrocytes in lacuna surrounded by an extracellular matrix strongly stained by type II collagen antibodies; (B) monolayer cultures of C1-derived adipocytes after 20 days of treatment with DEX and insulin: fat droplets stained with oil red O; (C) β-GP and AA-treated nodules at 15 days of osteogenic differentiation showing matrix mineralization stained by Von Kossa; (D) Toluidine blue staining of control nodules at day 50.

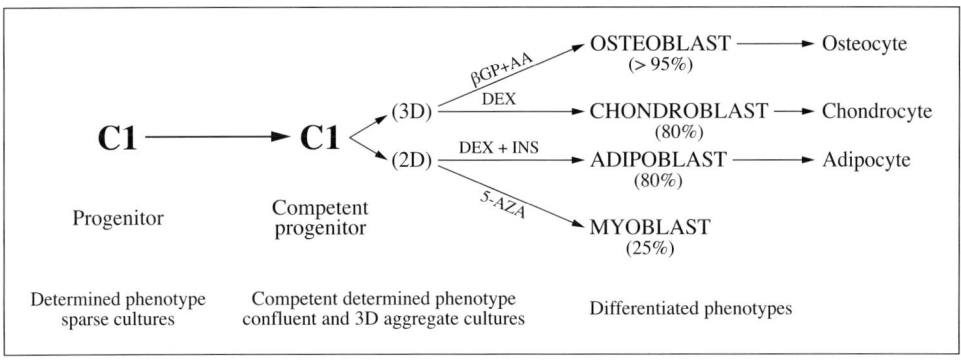

Figure 5. The different steps of C1 stem cell differentiation.

PTHRP, Ihh, Notch, Soxs) involved in the complex network of pathways leading to embryonic skeletal development (current work). These factors, together with time-dependent interactions with matrix components, may lead each of the intrinsic programs of the C1 progenitor (and in particular chondrogenesis) to proceed in a cell-autonomous way.

In summary, immortalization of pluripotent somatic stem cells through differentiation of ES or EC multipotential cells is aimed at bringing answers to fundamental question such as "which signalling pathways govern the entry and progression of a stem cell into a genetic differentiation program and thereafter control and coordinate the expression of specialized function of its differentiated progeny." Such an *in vitro* immortalizing approach to isolate clonal cell lines may complement *in vivo* analyses since it permits identification of signalling mechanisms controlling differentiation in an integrated and homogenous phenotypic context.

Despite the growing interest in the field of stem cells, little is still known about the genes driving the recruitment and implementation of lineage specific programs. In this context, screening for genes differentially expressed in lineage precursors and in ES/EC cells may allow for identification of markers of somatic stem cells for somatic gene therapy.

Our observations of the neuronal or mesoblastic cell lines indicate that upon recruitment by a unique set of paracrine factor(s), the cells acquire a defined identity and proceed in a self organizing way to develop an entire differentiation program. Possibly, the intrinsic commitment of stem cells renders them competent and self-sufficient to reconstitute, *in vitro*, a microenvironment favouring functional differentiation.

Every new differentiation model with proliferative and differentiative properties has potential fundamental and medical implications. Oncogene-dependent isolation of somatic stem cell lines precludes the use of the resulting immortalized clones for gene therapy. Nevertheless, immortalization strategies of multilineage stem cells from multipotential cells may prove useful in identifying how the interplay between intrinsic and extrinsic factors can recruit, restrict and specify the fate of a pluripotent stem cell.

Acknowledgments

This work was supported by grants from CNRS, ARC and CNP foundation. M.B. is recipient of a FNRS fellowship.

References

1. Kellermann O, Kelly F. Immortalization of early embryonic cell derivatives after transfer of Simian virus 40 early region into F9 teratocarcinoma cells. *Differentiation* 1986; 32: 74-81.
2. Kelly F, Boccara M. Susceptibility of teratocarcinoma cells to adenovirus type 2. *Nature* 1976; 262: 409-11.
3. Kellermann O, Buc-Caron MH, Gaillard J. Immortalization of precursors of endodermal, neuroectodermal, mesodermal lineages following the introduction of the SV40 early region into F9 cells. *Differentiation* 1987; 35: 197-205.
4. Buc MH, Launay JM, Lamblin D, Kellermann O. Serotonin uptake, storage and synthesis in a immortalized commited cell line derived from mouse teratocarcinoma. *Proc Natl Acad Sci USA* 1990; 87: 1922-6.
5. Kellermann O, Buc-Caron MH, Marie PJ, Lamblin D, Jacob F. An immortalized osteogenic cell line derived from mouse teratocarcinoma is able to mineralize *in vivo*. *J Cell Biol* 1990; 110: 123-32.
6. Mouillet-Richard S, Mutel V, Loric S, Tournois C, Launay JM, Kellermann O. Mutually-exclusive induction of the 1C11 neuroectodermal cell line towards fully functional serotoninergic or catecholaminergic differentiation programs. *J Biol Chem* 2000; 13: 9186-92.
7. Lauder JM. Neurotransmitters as growth regulatory signals: role of receptors and second messengers. *Trends Neurosci* 1993; 16: 233-40.

8. Bronner-Fraser M, Fraser SE. Differentiation of the vertebrate neural tube. *Curr Opin Cell Biol* 1997; 9: 885-91.
9. Wilkinson DG, Bhatt S, Chavrier P, Bravo R, Charnay P. Segment-specific expression of a zinc-finger gene in the developing nervous system of the mouse. *Nature* 1989; 337: 461-4.
10. Guillemot F, Joyner AL. Dynamic expression of the murine Achaete-scute homologue Mash-1 in the developing nervous system. *Mech Dev* 1993; 42: 171-85.
11. Ye W, Shimamura K, Rubenstein JL, Hynes MA, Rosenthal A. FGF and Shh signals control dopaminergic and serotoninergic cell fate in the anterior neural plate. *Cell* 1998; 93 (5): 755-66.
12. Kellermann O, Loric S, Maroteaux L, Launay JM. Sequential onset of three serotonin receptors during the serotoninergic differentiation of the 1C11 cell line. *Br J Pharmacol* 1996; 118: 1161-70.
13. Hyde CE, Bennett BA. Similar properties of fetal and adult amine transporters in the rat brain. *Brain Res* 1994; 646 (1): 118-23.
14. Jonakait GM, Markey KA, Goldstein M, Dreyfus CF, Black IB. Selective expression of high-affinity uptake of catecholamines by transiently catecholaminergic cells of the rat embryo: studies *in vivo* and *in vitro*. *Dev Biol* 1985; 108: 6-17.
15. Choi DS, Loric S, Colas JF, Callebert J, Rosay P, Kellermann O, Launay JM, Maroteaux L. The mouse 5-HT2B receptor, homologous subtype or species variant? *Behav Brain Res* 1996; 73: 253-7.
16. Hoyer D, Clarke DE, Fozard JR, Hartig PR, Martin GR, Mylecharane EJ, Saxena PR, Humphrey PP. International Union of Pharmacology classification of receptors for 5-hydroxytryptamine (Serotonin). *Pharmacol Rev* 1994; 46: 157-203.
17. Loric S, Maroteaux L, Kellermann O, Launay JM. Functional serotonin-2B receptors are expressed by a teratocarcinoma-derived cell line during serotoninergic differentiation. *Mol Pharmacol* 1995; 47: 458-66.
18. Launay JM, Birraux G, Bondoux D, Callebert J, Choi DS, Loric S, Maroteaux L. Ras involvement in signal transduction by the serotonin 5-HT2B receptor. *J Biol Chem* 1996; 271: 3141-7.
19. Manivet P, Mouillet-Richard S, Callebert J, Hosoda S, Maroteaux L, Kellermann O, Launay JM. PDZ-dependent activation of NO synthases by the serotonin-2B receptor. *J Biol Chem* 2000; 13: 9324-331.
20. Tournois C, Mutel V, Manivet P, Launay JM, Kellermann O. Crosstalk between 5-HT receptors in a serotoninergic cell line: involvement of arachidonic acid metabolism. *J Biol Chem* 1998; 273: 17498-503.
21. Aubin JE, Turksen K, Heersche JNM. Osteoblastic cell lineage. In: Noda M, ed. *Cellular and molecular biology of bone*. New York: Academic Press, 1993: 1-45.
22. Cancedda R, Cancedda FD, Castagnola P. Chondrocyte differentiation. *Int Rev Cytol* 1995; 159: 265-358.
23. Poliard A, Nifuji A, Lamblin D, Plee E, Forest C, Kellermann O. Controlled conversion of an immortalized mesodermal stem cell towards osteogenic, chondrogenic or adipogenic pathways. *J Cell Biol* 1995; 130: 1461-72.
24. Poliard A, Ronzière MC, Freyria AM, Lamblin D, Herbage D, Kellermann O. Lineage-dependent collagen expression and assembly by a tripotential mesoblastic cell line to the endstages of osteogenic, chondrogenic or adipogenic differentiation. *Exp Cell Res* 1999; 253: 385-95.
25. Poliard A, Lamblin D, Marie PJ, Buc-Caron MH, Kellermann O. Commitment of the teratocarcinoma-derived mesodermal clone C1 towards terminal osteogenic differentiation. *J Cell Sci* 1993; 106: 503-11.

Directed differentiation of dendritic cells from mouse embryonic stem cells: a novel tool for identifying targets for immunotherapy

Paul J. Fairchild[1], Frances A. Brook[2], Richard L. Gardner[2], Luis Graça[1], Victoria Strong[1], Yukiko Tone[1], Masahide Tone[1], Kathleen F. Nolan[1], Herman Waldmann[1]

[1] Sir William Dunn School of Pathology, University of Oxford, Oxford, United Kingdom
[2] Department of Zoology, University of Oxford, Oxford, United Kingdom

Summary – Dendritic cells (DC) form a diverse system of antigen presenting cells (APC) responsible for orchestrating the body's response to infection. As the only cell type capable of eliciting effector functions among antigen-naïve T cells, DC act at the very heart of the immune response, either driving immunity or securing a state of self-tolerance. Although DC hold promise as targets for immune intervention, the mechanisms responsible for defining the balance between these opposing forces currently remain obscure. While techniques for analysing differential gene expression have begun to identify novel DC-specific genes that may be involved, an approach to elucidating their function is presently lacking, due, primarily, to the resistance of primary DC to genetic modification. Given the propensity for genetic manipulation of embryonic stem (ES) cells and the potential for their directed differentiation *in vitro*, we have defined the culture conditions and growth factors required for their commitment to the DC lineage. Here we describe the derivation of long-term cultures of cells displaying the characteristics of immature DC, including the capacity to acquire and process foreign antigen for presentation to T cells. Exposure to inflammatory stimuli induces the terminal differentiation of these precursors causing them to adopt the morphology and surface phenotype of mature DC, capable of stimulating primary responses among allogeneic T cells. These findings pave the way for the rational design of DC lines competent to function in immunity, in which candidate genes have been over-expressed or functionally ablated. Exploration of the unique properties of such mutant DC may help define novel targets for intervention in the pathogenesis of immunologically-related disease.

A cardinal feature of the adaptive immune system is its inherent specificity for antigen, permitting the mounting of an immune response, designed to exploit the vulnerability of particular micro-organisms. Such specificity is achieved by the generation of vast repertoires of T and B lymphocytes, whose surface receptors for antigen show unparalleled conformational diversity: conservative estimates suggest the potential for synthesizing as many as 10^9 structural variants of both the T-cell receptor (TCR) and immunoglobulin molecules by the random rearrangement of the multiple gene segments that encode them. Only by expressing these receptors in a clonal fashion, may the adaptive immune system meet the challenge posed by the immense diversity of potential pathogens.

Although the evolutionary advantage conferred on higher vertebrates by adaptive immunity undoubtedly lies in its specificity, such advances create a number of logistic difficulties. Firstly, the probability that rare T cells, among such a vast repertoire, will encounter their cognate antigen purely by chance, is vanishingly small, requiring the intervention of a dedicated antigen presenting cell (APC) capable of delivering the components of pathogens to the relevant clones. Secondly, any system for generating diversity which relies on random gene rearrangement risks the emergence of cells with greater specificity for self proteins than foreign antigens, requiring their subsequent removal, functional silencing or active regulation in order to maintain self-tolerance. Both of these dilemmas have been resolved, in evolutionary terms, by a system of cells with unique properties: the dendritic cells.

The dendritic cell life cycle

Dendritic cells (DC) form an extensive network of bone marrow-derived APC which are disseminated widely throughout the body, occupying both the interstitial tissues and lymphoid organs [1]. In contrast to other populations of professional APC, the elaborate life cycle of the DC ensures that the processes of antigen acquisition and its subsequent presentation to T cells, remain spatially and temporally separate [2] *(figure 1)*. Within interstitial tissues, DC appear arrested at a stage of immaturity, associated with a sentinel function. Here, they display a voracity for antigen uptake strongly reminiscent of the macrophage (MØ): indeed, immature DC share many of the functional and phenotypic properties of MØ including their propensity for phagocytosis and expression of surface markers such as F4/80, FcR and CD11b.

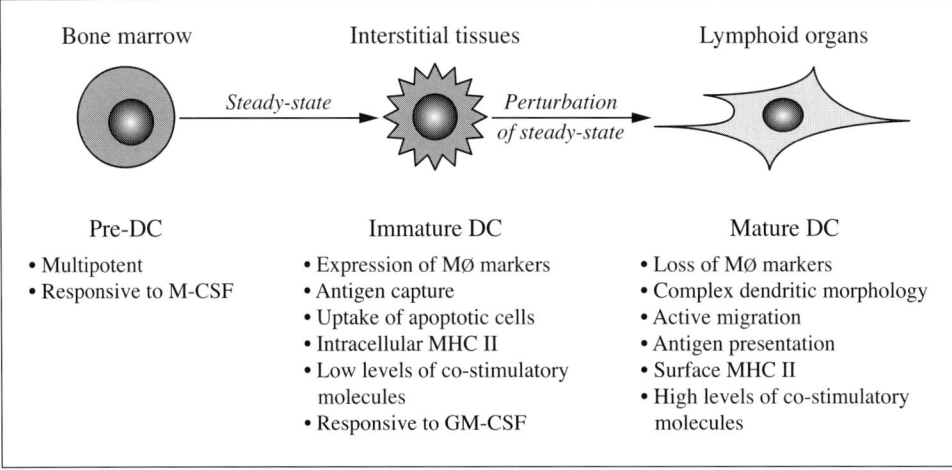

Figure 1. Schematic representation of DC differentiation from committed progenitors in the bone marrow. Under steady state conditions, pre-DC seed interstitial tissues where they give rise to a population of immature DC displaying the propensity for antigen acquisition, indicative of a sentinel function. Perturbation of the steady state through infection is responsible for driving maturation of DC, which migrate to secondary lymphoid organs where they present antigen to naïve T cells.

Despite these similarities, the defining feature of DC is their capacity to respond to inflammatory stimuli [3] and a variety of bacterial and viral products [4], by initiating a coordinated series of events, culminating in their maturation. During the accompanying changes, DC relinquish any preoccupation with antigen capture, favouring, instead, its presentation at the cell surface as peptide fragments bound to products of the major histocompatibility complex (MHC) [5]. Furthermore, the up-regulation of co-stimulatory molecules such as CD40, CD80 and CD86, in concert with TCR ligands [6], confers to the DC the unique capacity to activate naïve T cells. Rather than presenting their cargo of antigen at the site of infection, however, DC migrate *via* the afferent lymphatics to the spleen and draining lymph nodes where they interdigitate within the T cell areas [7]. By clustering with large numbers of T cells, DC efficiently peruse the repertoire, identifying those rare clones specific for the antigens they harbour and stimulating their clonal expansion to meet the challenge of infection. Although the efflux of DC progenitors from the bone marrow occurs constitutively under steady state conditions, it is the perturbation of the steady state through infection which is responsible for driving the terminal maturation of DC and initiating the primary immune response *(figure 1)*.

Dendritic cells and self-tolerance

That DC are uniquely capable of activating inexperienced T cells helps define the conceptual limits of self-tolerance. The minimal intervention necessary for avoiding autoreactivity requires the elimination of T cells specific for the self peptides presented by DC: self components presented solely by other APC pose little threat to the integrity of the host, due to their impotence in triggering a primary response. It is, therefore, unsurprising that DC fulfil the complementary roles of antigen presentation for both immunity and self-tolerance.

The tolerogenic credentials of the DC are best illustrated within the thymus, the initial site of T-cell repertoire selection. Here, the recognition of self antigen results in the apoptosis of autoreactive T cells and their deletion from the nascent repertoire [8, 9]. While the specialised function of thymic DC has been appreciated for some years, recent evidence has suggested that such tolerogenic potential is not confined to the thymus but is of equal importance within the periphery, where challenges to the tolerant state must be actively opposed. Indeed, constitutive pathways of DC migration have begun to emerge, devoted to the transport of apoptotic debris from interstitial tissues, such as the gut, to the draining lymph nodes [10, 11], the presentation of self components in such a non-inflammatory context, most likely reinforcing self-tolerance [12, 13]. Interestingly, it may be these same pathways that are accessed therapeutically by the oral administration of antigen, widely claimed to lead to a state of functional tolerance [14]. Nevertheless, reports that the oral route of exposure to antigen may also prime T cells under some circumstances [15, 16] and the discovery that DC migrating from the gut may present such antigens in an immunogenic fashion [17], emphasises the delicate balance that DC achieve between tolerance and immunity [18, 19] while highlighting how little is currently known of the parameters regulating these opposing forces.

Dendritic cells and prospects for immunotherapy

Despite these uncertainties, the involvement of DC at the very genesis of all immune responses, whether protective or pathogenic, provides unparalleled opportunities to influence the outcome of antigen presentation for therapeutic gain. Consequently, DC have become the focus of novel strategies for immune intervention, aimed either at enhancing responsiveness for the purpose of vaccination, or limiting the extent of its impact, when mounted inappropriately. Murine DC exposed *ex vivo* to non-viable *Chlamydia* have, for instance, been shown to initiate a powerful immune response upon readministration *in vivo*, conferring on recipients protection from subsequent infection [20]. Such findings suggest the use of DC to be effective in the elimination of intracellular parasites that have proven resistant to conventional approaches to vaccination. The adjuvanticity of DC, harnessed in such experiments, has been further exploited to selectively undermine the fragile state of tolerance to self components expressed by certain transformed tissues, thereby eliciting anti-tumour immunity [21]. Pulsing DC with tumour lysates, whole tumour RNA [22], or synthetic peptides derived from known tumour-specific antigens [23, 24], have proven effective strategies for achieving the regression of solid tumour masses [23] as well as established secondary metastases [25].

Although our understanding of the tolerogenic properties of DC in peripheral tissues is currently in its infancy, prospects for their use in ameliorating allograft rejection or taming ongoing autoimmune responses, remain an appealing possibility with at least some experimental support [26]. The administration of populations of immature donor-derived DC, devoid of co-stimulatory molecules, has achieved modest prolongation of graft survival in rodents [27], which may be potentiated by the prevention of their maturation *in vivo*, through the blockade of CD40 ligation [28]. Furthermore, the intrathymic injection of allopeptide-pulsed DC has been shown to result in indefinite cardiac allograft survival [29]. Likewise, the intravenous administration of thymic DC, pulsed with an autoantigenic epitope of myelin basic protein, prevented the onset of experimental autoimmune encephalomyelitis (EAE) in a susceptible strain of rat [30]. Although the mechanisms involved appear primarily deletional, the ability of DC to establish more robust forms of tolerance associated with active regulation, has been suggested in an animal model of diabetes. DC isolated from lymph nodes draining the pancreas of female NOD mice were able to adoptively transfer resistance to the onset of diabetes. The transfer of lymph node cells from such mice to secondary recipients likewise conferred protection from the infusion of a diabetogenic inoculum, observations which are consistent with the emergence of a population of regulatory T cells [31].

Hurdles to the therapeutic exploitation of dendritic cells

Although the success of these studies has heightened expectations for the future application of DC within the clinic, a number of hurdles must be overcome before such hopes may be realised. Details such as the most appropriate source of precursors from which to culture autologous human DC, the most effective route of administration and the development of substitutes for fetal calf serum, required for their maintenance *in vitro*, still remain unresolved [32]. Beyond these various logistics, however, lie a number of more fundamental issues, the most significant being our current lack of insight into the molecular basis of DC function and the balance they define between tolerance and immunity. Such uncertainty prevents their use in clinical trials with any degree of confidence, since the potential for inadvertently inducing tolerance to tumour antigens or enhancing immunity to autoantigenic epitopes remains a serious concern, threatening to exacerbate pre-existing disease.

Although the advent of powerful techniques for the analysis of differential gene expression has begun to uncover many novel DC-specific genes whose products may illuminate the dynamic between tolerance and immunity [33], elucidation of their function has proven the rate-limiting step in the study of DC biology. This inertia emanates from the remarkable resistance of primary DC to genetic modification and their short life span following terminal maturation *in vitro*, greatly diminishing the appeal of any such attempts. These limitations have been partly circumvented by the generation of DC lines from mice [34-36] which appear more amenable to genetic intervention [37]; nevertheless, their apparent arrest at an early stage of the DC life cycle [38] limits prospects for investigating gene function at the terminal stages of maturation, associated with immunogenicity. Furthermore, the need for retroviral transformation to confer immortality on some of these lines [34, 35] risks the introduction of experimental artifacts, while inevitably restricting their use *in vivo*.

It is largely as a result of these experimental obstacles that the production of mice deficient in the gene of interest, by means of knockout technology, currently remains the most definitive approach to assessing gene function. Nevertheless, the establishment of such strains is both time-consuming and labour-intensive and is, therefore, inappropriate as a high-throughput system. Furthermore, the inability to apply such technology to humans has done little to demolish the species barrier, making it difficult to confirm the function of the human homologues of any promising new genes.

Overcoming the impass: a novel source of dendritic cells

Given the unparalleled potential that DC offer for the treatment of immunologically-based disease, we have adopted a distinctive approach to their study with the potential for resolving a number of the limitations of existing strategies. The availability of pluripotent embryonic stem (ES) cell lines with proven capacity for differentiation *in vitro* suggests the potential for their directed differentiation towards the DC lineage. Such an approach would combine the convenience and flexibility of a DC line, with the distinct advantages of untransformed, primary DC. Furthermore, the very same propensity for genetic manipulation that has fuelled the revolution of knockout technology, might be harnessed for the rational design of DC bearing a desired, mutant phenotype.

To this end, we have developed a panel of ES cell lines from the delayed-implanting blastocysts of CBA/Ca mice [38], one of which (ESF116) was found to be karyotypically male and germline competent upon its reintroduction into blastocysts from a random-bred albino strain of mouse (PO mice: Pathology Oxford): from a total of 19 progeny, 8 chimeras were obtained, 2 of which were found to transmit the CBA genome through the germline. ESF116 could be cultured undifferentiated on monolayers of mitotically-inactivated embryonic fibroblasts or on gelatinized flasks in medium supplemented with recombinant leukaemia inhibitory factor (LIF). Upon their culture at low density on bacteriological plastic, however, ESF116 rapidly formed both simple and cystic embryoid bodies (EB), known to provide an effective microenvironment for supporting the early stages of hematopoiesis [39, 40]. Although various populations of leukocytes have been reported to develop from such cultures, including mast cells, Mø [41], T cells [42] and B cells [43], the derivation of DC has not previously been described.

EB were, therefore, plated onto tissue culture plastic in medium supplemented with conditioned media and growth factors implicated in DC ontogeny. After overnight culture, the majority of EB adhered to the substrate and produced discrete colonies of stromal cells emigrating outwards in a radial fashion *(figure 2a)*. Within 4 to 5 days, cells with distinctive dendritic morphology began to appear, the phenotype and function of which identified them unequivocally as DC [44]. These ES cell-derived DC (esDC) were consistently confined to the very perimeter of colonies, up to 95% of which proved permissive. Furthermore, their appearance was neither strain-dependent nor confined to EB from ESF116, since two further lines, ESF75, derived from C57Bl/6 mice, and another line of CBA origin (ESF99), likewise supported their growth.

The distinctive distribution of esDC from all three lines revealed a clear demarcation between areas of the underlying stroma capable of supporting their development and those that consistently failed to do so *(figure 2b, asterisk)*. Importantly, esDC that had originated around the very edge of colonies formed large clusters reminiscent of immature DC derived from cultures of bone marrow (bmDC) [45]; over the ensuing 8 to 10 days, cells released from these clusters seeded uncolonized areas of tissue culture plastic, where they expanded rapidly in number *(figure 2c)*, forming long-term cultures of lightly adherent cells that could be harvested routinely by gentle pipetting. Individual EB micromanipulated into the wells of 24 well plates, generated, on average, approximately 4×10^5 esDC within 14 days. Repeated harvesting of this population with a 6 to 7 day periodicity showed their propensity to rapidly regenerate. Nevertheless, the gradual and consistent decline in yields with time *(figure 3)* suggested they had lost the potential for self-renewal, indicative of *bona fide* stem cells, but displayed, instead, the vast, yet finite, proliferative capacity normally attributed to populations of transit amplifying cells. Despite retaining some of the characteristics of early precursors, however, these cells displayed the morphology and ultrastructure of immature DC, including numerous cytoplasmic processes and the distribution of mitochondria, vacuoles and endocytic structures characteristic of bmDC [45] *(figure 2d)*.

Interestingly, visualisation of esDC by electron microscopy revealed occasional cells that had phagocytosed whole apoptotic bodies, derived from their local microenvironment *(figure 2e)*. The capacity for phagocytosis of apoptotic cells is a property shared by Mø and immature DC and constitutes a route of antigen acquisition that has been variously linked with the phenomena of cross-priming and cross-tolerance [13, 46]. Consistent with the ability of esDC to present captured antigens to T cells in a classic MHC-restricted fashion, cells pulsed with whole hen eggwhite lysozyme (HEL) stimulated the dose-dependent release of interleukin 2 (IL-2) by an antigen-specific T cell hybridoma *(Table I)*. The surface phenotype of esDC confirmed their arrest at an

Directed differentiation of dendritic cells from mouse embryonic stem cells

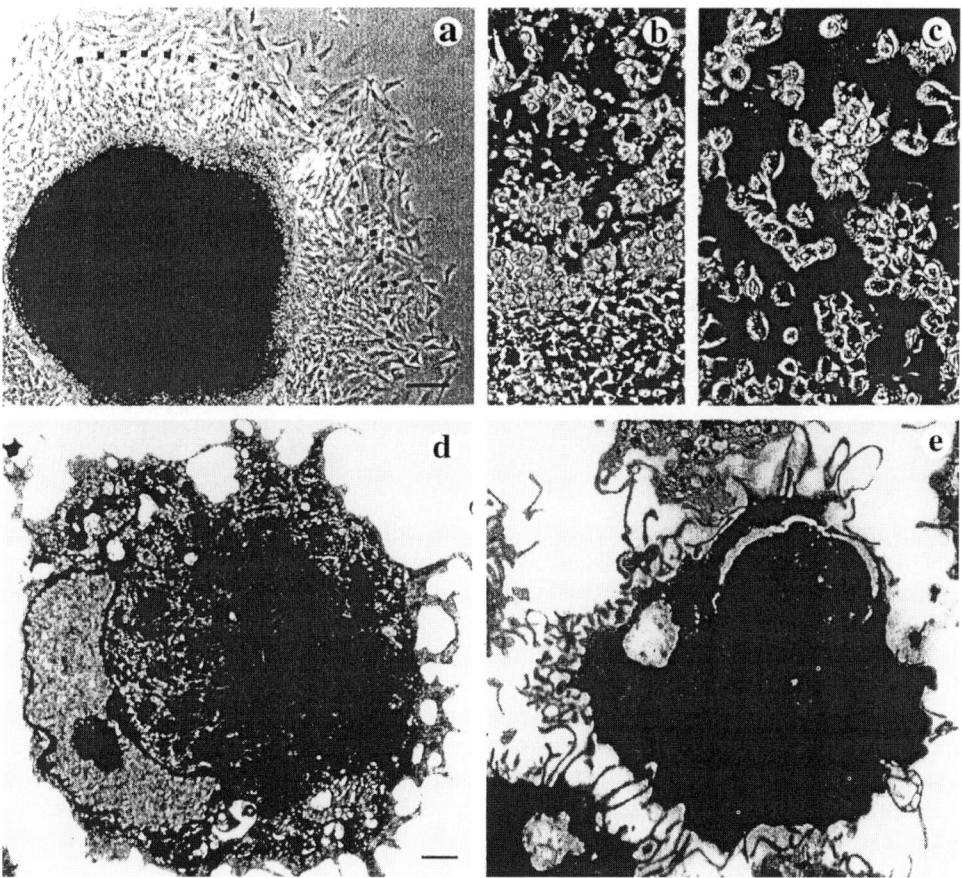

Figure 2. Derivation and ultrastructure of esDC. (a) Low power phase contrast micrograph of a single EB 48 hr after culturing on tissue culture plastic, showing the radial emigration of stromal cells. The broken line indicates the approximate location of esDC that begin to appear 48 hr later. (b) The early emergence of esDC, showing the clear demarcation between areas of stroma supporting their development and those that fail to do so (asterisk). (c) An established culture of esDC growing on areas of the culture vessel free of underlying stroma. (d-e) Transmission EM micrographs of immature esDC, showing characteristic dendritic morphology (d) and the propensity for phagocytosis of apoptotic cells (e). The bars represent 100 μm (a), 50 μm (b and c) and 1 μm (d and e).

Table I. Properties of esDC compared with other populations of APC.

Property	Mø	esDC	bmDC	Splenic DC
High proliferative capacity	-	++	+	-
Responsiveness to M-CSF	+	-	-	-
NO secretion	++	++	+	-
Phagocytosis	++	+	+	-
Endocytosis	++	++	++	-
Antigen processing	++	++	++	-
Presentation of acquired antigen	+	++	++	++
Stimulation of naïve T cells	-	++	++	++

Table II. Surface phenotype of esDC compared with other APC.

Surface marker	Mø	Immature esDC	Mature esDC	Immature bmDC	Splenic DC
CD44	+	++	++	++	++
CD45	+	+	+	+	+
MHC I	+	+	+	+	++
MHC II	±	±	++	+	++
CD11c	-	-	+	+	+
CD40	±	-	+	-	++
CD54	±	+	++	+	++
CD80	±	±	++	+	++
CD86	±	-	++	±	++
RANK	-	+	+	+	+
F4/80	++	+	±	+	-
CD11b	++	+	±	+	-
FcγR	++	+	±	+	-

immature stage, closely associated with antigen acquisition. These cells displayed only low levels of MHC class II molecules, due to their retention within intracellular compartments, and were relatively deficient in expression of the costimulatory molecules CD40, CD54, CD80 and CD86 *(Table II)*. Interestingly, their expression of the scavenger receptor, mannose receptor and the macrophage markers F4/80 and CD11b reinforced the same close allegiance to Mø, evident among cultures of immature bmDC. Indeed, exposure of esDC to lipopolysaccharide (LPS) induced the release of substantial quantities of nitric oxide (NO) that could be enhanced by interferon-γ (IFN-γ) and abrogated by the addition of N^G-monomethyl-L-arginine (NMMA), a specific inhibitor of inducible nitric oxide synthase (iNOS) *(figure 4)*. This propensity for NO release is a hallmark of Mø, shared by bmDC *(figure 4)*, but absent from mature populations purified from secondary lymphoid organs such as the spleen.

Despite their evident similarities with Mø, highly-enriched populations of esDC failed to respond to macrophage colony stimulating factor (M-CSF) either by proliferation or detectable changes in their morphology and phenotype, suggesting they had already diverged from progenitors committed to the macrophage lineage. Consistent with this conclusion, esDC were capable of clustering with naïve, allogeneic T cells and inducing their blastogenesis and proliferation *(figure 5a, Table I)*, the defining characteristic of DC. Furthermore, interaction with T cells led to the terminal maturation of esDC which could be mimicked by their exposure to LPS: cells treated in this way adopted the veiled appearance of mature DC *(figure 5b)* and strongly up-regulated MHC class II, the DC-specific marker CD11c, and the co-stimulatory molecules CD40, CD54, CD80 and CD86 *(Table II)*. In addition to down-regulating macrophage markers *(Table II)*, mature esDC showed the ability to stimulate naïve, allogeneic T cells with a potency 10 times greater than their immature counterparts.

The application of esDC to immunotherapy

Identification of the culture conditions and growth factors required for the directed differentiation of DC from mouse ES cells offers a number of distinct advantages to

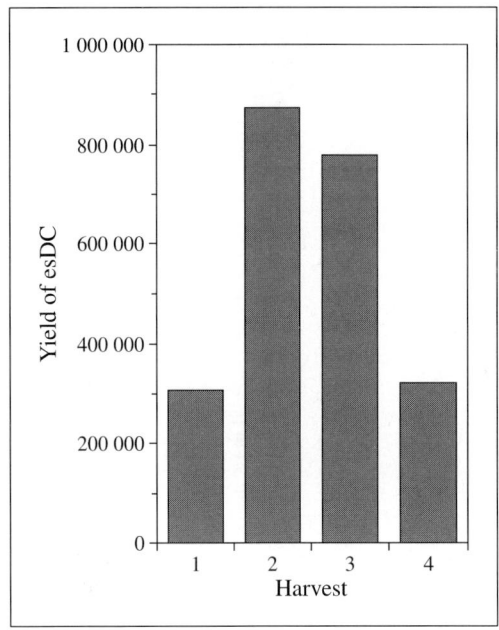

Figure 3. Typical yields of esDC from a single EB, harvested on 4 successive occasions, at intervals of 6 to 7 days. Numbers on the abscissa refer to each of these 4 events.

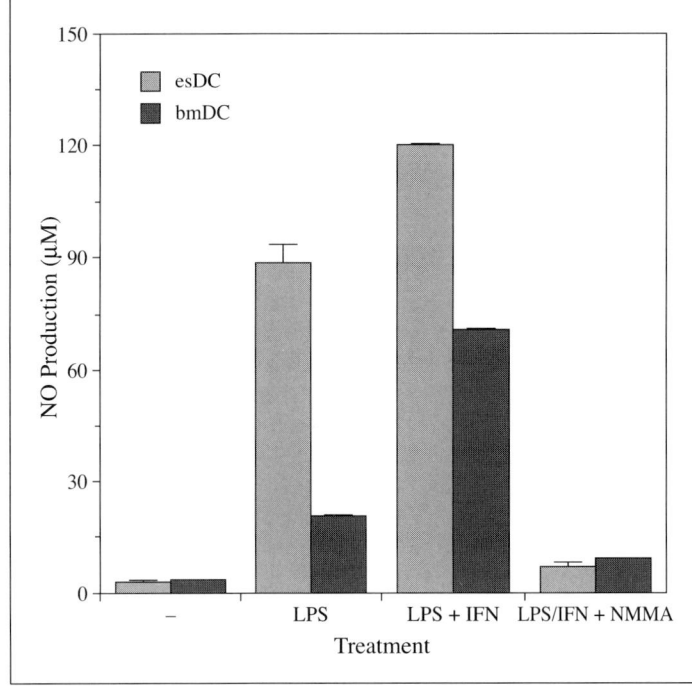

Figure 4. Comparison of NO secretion by esDC and bmDC. DC derived from ES cells fail to secrete NO under normal circumstances but release high quantities when challenged with LPS +/- interferon-γ (IFN). This secretion of NO may be abrogated by the addition of NMMA, a specific inhibitor of iNOS.

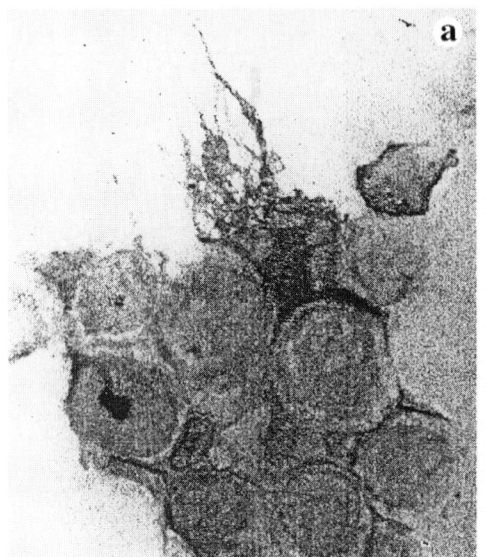 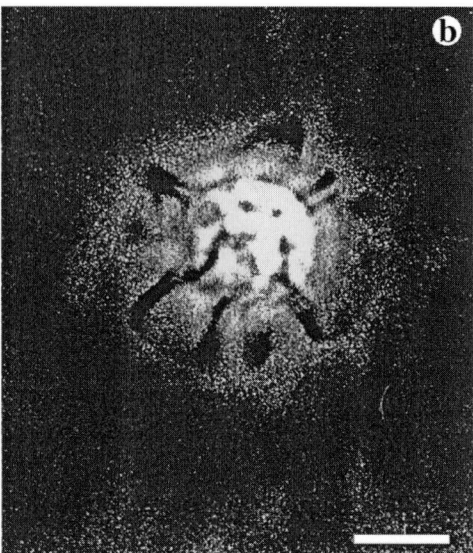

Figure 5. Maturation of esDC. (a) When co-cultured with naïve, allogeneic T cells, esDC form large clusters, inducing the activation and blastogenesis of alloreactive cells. Conversely, the interaction with T cells is a powerful stimulus for esDC maturation inducing their upregulation of MHC class II (brown staining). (b) Exposure to LPS acts as a surrogate stimulus for maturation of esDC which acquire the veiled appearance of mature cells after overnight culture. The bar represents 5 μm.

the study of DC biology. These cells form long-term cultures, which are phenotypically stable with time, failing to undergo the progressive maturation evident among cultures of bmDC, yet retaining the capacity to mature upon exposure to the appropriate stimuli. Given that a single EB may sustain the growth of many millions of esDC, and that a single passage of the parent ES cell line may yield thousands of viable EB, the number of available cells has never, in our experience, proved limiting. Undoubtedly the most important facet of the system we have developed, however, is the potential for genetic modification at the ES cell stage, raising prospects for the rational design of primary DC, bearing a desired, mutant phenotype.

Although a number of approaches have been employed for the introduction of heterologous genes into populations of primary DC, each is limited in its application. The use of mRNA has, for example, proven successful [47], but represents, at best, a transient expression system. Ballistic approaches have likewise proven effective [48] but transfection efficiencies may be low, while the physical trauma associated with such an approach may adversely affect DC function. Perhaps the most widely exploited technique has been the use of adenoviral vectors. Nevertheless, with transduction efficiencies frequently reported to be as low as 30%, the need for sorting those cells of the desired phenotype becomes imperative. Furthermore, the exposure of DC to adenovirus mimics the initial encounter between DC and infectious microorganisms, frequently inducing their terminal maturation [49]: while maturation greatly reduces the life span of the resulting mutants, it also prevents the investigation of gene function during the earliest stages of the DC life cycle. Clearly, by smuggling heterologous genes into esDC at the stem cell stage, many of these hurdles may be overcome. Furthermore, while each of the conventional strategies to genetic modification permits the over-expression of desired genes, the description of protocols for the generation of ES cells in which both alleles of a given gene have been functionally ablated [50], uniquely harnesses the additional potential of knockout technology for the investigation of gene function in DC.

We envisage, therefore, that novel DC-specific genes that have begun to emerge from studies of differential gene expression may be either functionally ablated or over-expressed in ES cells, permitting the generation of "designer" DC with previously-unexplored properties *(figure 6)*. Such an approach may help identify novel targets for immune intervention, with the ultimate prospect of modifying DC function *in vivo* as a way of reinforcing self-tolerance or enhancing immunity. Most significantly, however, the recent derivation of ES cells from human blastocysts [51] and their proven capacity for somatic differentiation *in vitro* [52] may extend our approach to the study of the human homologues of candidate genes, bridging the species barrier and bringing DC-based immunotherapy one step closer to the clinic.

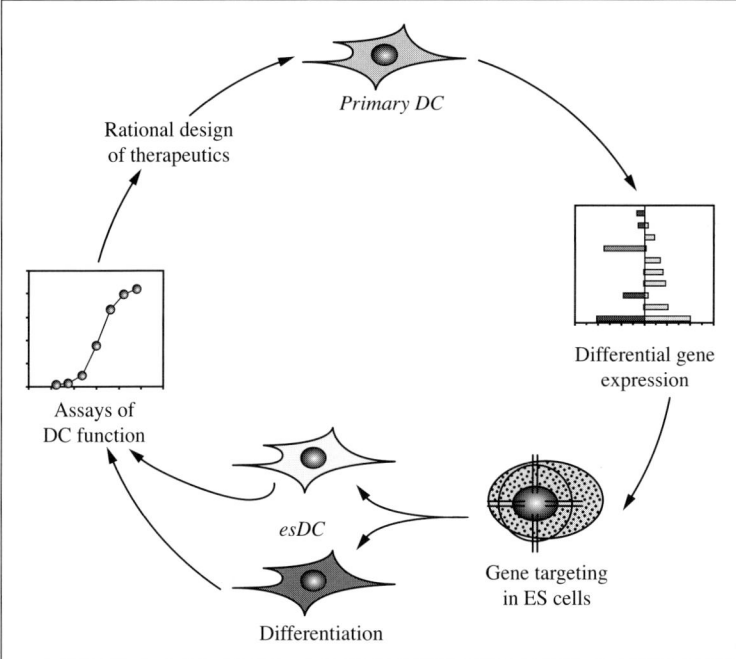

Figure 6. Schematic diagram showing the likely application of esDC to the development of novel strategies for immunotherapy. Studies of differential gene expression among populations of primary DC have begun to uncover DC-specific genes of unknown function. Gene targeting strategies, performed on the parent ES cell line, may allow the differentiation of esDC either overexpressing or functionally deficient in the gene of interest. Elucidation of the properties of such "designer" DC in established assays may permit the identification of targets for therapeutic intervention, raising the prospect of influencing the function of primary DC *in situ*.

Acknowledgements

This work was supported by a Programme Grant from the Medical Research Council (UK). VS is the recipient of a Philip Walker studentship. RLG acknowledges the support of the Royal Society, FAB the support of the British Diabetic Association and LG the Gulbenkian Foundation and the Portuguese Foundation for Science and Technology for the provision of a scholarship.

References

1. Banchereau J, Steinman RM. Dendritic cells and the control of immunity. *Nature* 1998; 392: 245-52.
2. Mellman I, Turley SJ, Steinman RM. Antigen processing for amateurs and professionals. *Trends Cell Biol* 1998; 8: 231-7.
3. Cella M, Engering A, Pinet V, Pieters J, Lanzavecchia A. Inflammatory stimuli induce accumulation of MHC class II complexes on dendritic cells. *Nature* 1997; 388: 782-7.
4. Rescigno M, Granucci F, Citterio S, Foti M, Ricciardi-Castagnoli P. Coordinated events in bacteria-induced DC maturation. *Immunol Today* 1999; 20: 200-3.
5. Pierre P, Turley SJ, Gatti E, Hull M, Meltzer J, Mirza A, Inaba K, Steinman RM, Mellman I. Developmental regulation of MHC class II transport in mouse dendritic cells. *Nature* 1997; 388: 787-92.
6. Turley SJ, Inaba K, Garrett WS, Ebersold M, Unternaehrer J, Steinman RM, Mellman I. Transport of peptide-MHC class II complexes in developing dendritic cells. *Science* 2000; 288: 522-7.
7. Ingulli E, Mondino A, Khoruts A, Jenkins MK. In vivo detection of dendritic cell antigen presentation to $CD4^+$ T cells. *J Exp Med* 1997; 185: 2133-41.
8. Fairchild PJ, Austyn JM. Thymic dendritic cells: phenotype and function. *Int Rev Immunol* 1990; 6: 187-96.
9. Ardavin C. Thymic dendritic cells. *Immunol Today* 1997; 18: 350-61.
10. Huang FP, Platt N, Wykes M, Major JR, Powell TJ, Jenkins CD, MacPherson GG. A discrete subpopulation of dendritic cells transports apoptotic intestinal epithelial cells to T cell areas of mesenteric lymph nodes. *J Exp Med* 2000; 191: 435-43.
11. Vezys V, Olson S, Lefrançois L. Expression of intestine-specific antigen reveals novel pathways of CD8 T cell tolerance induction. *Immunity* 2000; 12: 505-14.
12. Steinman RM, Turley S, Mellman I, Inaba K. The induction of tolerance by dendritic cells that have captured apoptotic cells. *J Exp Med* 2000; 191: 411-6.
13. Heath WR, Kurts C, Miller JFAP, Carbone FR. Cross tolerance: a pathway for inducing tolerance to peripheral tissue antigens. *J Exp Med* 1998; 188: 1549-53.
14. Weiner HL, Friedman A, Miller A, Khoury SJ, al Sabbagh A, Santos L, Sayegh M, Nussenblatt RB, Trentham DE, Hafler DA. Oral tolerance: immunologic mechanisms and treatment of animal and human organ-specific autoimmune diseases by oral administration of autoantigens. *Annu Rev Immunol* 1994; 12: 809-37.
15. Blanas E, Carbone FR, Allison J, Miller JFAP, Heath WR. Induction of autoimmune diabetes by oral administration of autoantigen. *Science* 1996; 274: 1707-9.
16. Blanas E, Davey GM, Carbone FR, Heath WR. A bone marrow-derived APC in the gut-associated lymphoid tissue captures oral antigens and presents then to both $CD4^+$ and $CD8^+$ T cells. *J Immunol* 2000; 164: 2890-6.
17. Liu LM, MacPherson GG. Antigen acquisition by DC: Intestinal DC acquire antigen administered orally and can prime naive T cells *in vivo*. *J Exp Med* 1993; 177: 1299-307.
18. Finkelman FD, Lees A, Birnbaum R, Gause WC, Morris SC. Dendritic cells present antigen *in vivo* in a tolerogenic or immunogenic fashion. *J Immunol* 1996; 157: 1406-14.
19. Thomson AW, Lu L, Steptoe RJ, Starzl TE. Dendritic cells and the balance between transplant tolerance and immunity. In: Banchereau J, Dodet B, Schwartz R, Trannoy E, eds. *Immune tolerance*. Paris: Elsevier, 1996: 173-85.

20. Su H, Messer R, Whitmire W, Fischer E, Portis JC, Caldwell HD. Vaccination against Chlamydial genital tract infection after immunization with dendritic cells pulsed *ex vivo* with nonviable *Chlamydiae*. *J Exp Med* 1998; 188: 809-18.
21. Fong L, Engleman EG. Dendritic cells in cancer immunotherapy. *Annu Rev Immunol* 2000; 18: 245-73.
22. Ashley DM, Faiola B, Nair S, Hale LP, Bigner DD, Gilboa E. Bone marrow-generated dendritic cells pulsed with tumor extracts or tumor RNA induce antitumor immunity against central nervous system tumors. *J Exp Med* 1997; 186: 1177-82.
23. Mayordomo JI, Zorina T, Storkus WJ, Zitvogel L, Celluzi C, Falo LD, Melief CJ, Ildstad ST, Kast WM, Deleo AB, Lotze MT. Bone marrow derived DC pulsed with synthetic tumour peptides elicit protective and therapeutic antitumour immunity. *Nature Med* 1995; 1: 1297-302.
24. Celluzzi CM, Mayordomo JI, Storkus WJ, Lotze MT, Falo LD. Peptide-pulsed DC induce antigen-specific, CTL-mediated protective tumor immunity. *J Exp Med* 1996; 183: 283-7.
25. Gong J, Chen D, Kashiwaba M, Kufe D. Induction of antitumour activity by immunization with fusions of dendritic and carcinoma cells. *Nature Med* 1997; 3: 558-61.
26. Fairchild PJ, Waldmann H. Dendritic cells and prospects for transplantation tolerance. *Cur Opin Immunol* 2000; 12: 528-35.
27. Fu F, Li Y, Qian S, Lu L, Chambers F, Starzl TE, Fung JJ, Thomson AW. Costimulatory molecule-deficient dendritic cell progenitors (MHC class II$^+$, B7-1^{dim}, B7-2$^-$) prolong cardiac allograft survival in non-immunosuppressed recipients. *Transplantation* 1996; 62: 659-65.
28. Lu L, Li W, Fu F, Chambers FG, Qian S, Fung JJ, Thomson AW. Blockade of the CD40-CD40 ligand pathway potentiates the capacity of donor-derived dendritic cell progenitors to induce long-term cardiac allograft survival. *Transplantation* 1997; 64: 1808-15.
29. Garrovillo M, Ali A, Oluwole SF. Indirect allorecognition in acquired thymic tolerance: induction of donor-specific tolerance to rat cardiac allografts by allopeptide-pulsed host dendritic cells. *Transplantation* 1999; 68: 1827-34.
30. Khoury SJ, Gallon L, Chen W, Betres K, Russell ME, Hancock WW, Carpenter CB, Sayegh MH, Weiner HL. Mechanisms of acquired thymic tolerance in EAE: Thymic dendritic-enriched cells induce specific peripheral T cell unresponsiveness *in vivo*. *J Exp Med* 1995; 182: 357-66.
31. Clare-Salzler MJ, Brooks J, Chai A, Van Herle K, Anderson C. Prevention of diabetes in nonobese diabetic mice by dendritic cell transfer. *J Clin Invest* 1992; 90: 741-8.
32. Girolomoni G, Ricciardi-Castagnoli P. Dendritic cells hold promise for immunotherapy. *Immunol Today* 1997; 18: 102-4.
33. Hashimoto S, Suzuki T, Dong HY, Nagai S, Yamazaki N, Matsushima K. Serial analysis of gene expression in human monocyte-derived dendritic cells. *Blood* 1999; 94: 845-52.
34. Paglia P, Girolomoni G, Robbiati F, Granucci F, Ricciardi-Castagnoli P. Immortalized dendritic cell line fully competent in antigen presentation initiates primary T cell responses *in vivo*. *J Exp Med* 1993; 178: 1893-901.
35. Girolomoni G, Lutz MB, Pastore S, Assmann CU, Cavani A, Ricciardi-Castagnoli P. Establishment of a cell line with features of early dendritic cell precursors from fetal mouse skin. *Eur J Immunol* 1995; 25: 2163-9.
36. Xu S, Ariizumi K, Caceres-Dittmar G, Edelbaum D, Hashimoto K, Bergstresser PR, Takashima A. Successive generation of antigen-presenting dendritic cell lines from murine epidermis. *J Immunol* 1995; 154: 2697-705.
37. Gaspari C, Rescigno M, Granucci F, Citterio S, Matyszak MK, Sciurpi MT, Lanfrancone L, Ricciardi-Castagnoli P. Retroviral gene transfer, rapid selection, and maintenance of the immature phenotype in mouse dendritic cells. *J Leuko Biol* 1999; 66: 263-7.
38. Brook FA, Gardner RL. The origin and efficient derivation of embryonic stem cells in the mouse. *Proc Natl Acad Sci USA* 1997; 94: 5709-12.
39. Keller GM. *In vitro* differentiation of embryonic stem cells. *Cur Opin Cell Biol* 1995; 7: 862-9.
40. Snodgrass HR, Schmitt RM, Bruyns E. Embryonic stem cells and *in vitro* haematopoiesis. *J Cell Biochem* 1992; 49: 225-30.
41. Wiles MV, Keller G. Multiple hematopoietic lineages develop from ES cells in culture. *Development* 1991; 111: 259-67.
42. Gutierrez-Ramos JC, Palacios R. *In vitro* differentiation of embryonic stem cells into lymphocyte precursors able to generate T and B lymphocytes *in vivo*. *Proc Natl Acad Sci USA* 1992; 89: 9171-5.
43. Cho SK, Webber TD, Carlyle JR, Nakano T, Lewis SM, Zuniga-Pflucker JC. Functional characterization of B lymphocytes generated *in vitro* from ES cells. *Proc Natl Acad Sci USA* 1999; 96: 9797-802.

44. Fairchild PJ, Brook FA, Gardner RL, Graça L, Strong V, Tone Y, Tone M, Nolan KF, Waldmann H. Directed differentiation of dendritic cells from mouse embryonic stem cells. *Curr Biol* 2000; 10: 1515-8.
45. Inaba K, Inaba M, Romani N, Aya H, Deguchi M, Ikehara S, Muramatsu S, Steinman RM. Generation of large numbers of dendritic cells from mouse bone marrow cultures supplemented with GM-CSF. *J Exp Med* 1992; 176: 1693-702.
46. Albert ML, Sauter B, Bhardwaj N. Dendritic cells acquire antigen from apoptotic cells and induce class I-restricted CTLs. *Nature* 1998; 392: 86-9.
47. Boczkowski D, Nair SK, Snyder D, Gilboa E. Dendritic cells pulsed with RNA are potent antigen-presenting cells *in vitro* and *in vivo*. *J Exp Med* 1996; 184: 465-72.
48. Matsue H, Matsue K, Walters M, Okumura K, Yagita H, Takashima A. Induction of antigen-specific immunosuppression by CD95L cDNA-transfected "killer" dendritic cells. *Nature Med* 1999; 5: 930-7.
49. Sonderbye L, Feng S, Yacoubian S, Buehler H, Ahsan N, Mulligan R, Langhoff E. *In vivo* and *in vitro* modulation of immune stimulatory capacity of primary dendritic cells by adenovirus-mediated gene transduction. *Exp Clin Immunogenet* 1998; 15: 100-11.
50. Mortensen RM, Conner DA, Chao S, Geisterfer-Lowrance AA, Seidman JG. Production of homozygous mutant ES cells with a single targeting construct. *Mol Cell Biol* 1992; 12: 2391-5.
51. Thomson JA, Itskovitz-Eldor J, Shapiro SS, Waknitz MA, Swiergiel JJ, Marshall VS, Jones JM. Embryonic stem cell lines derived from human blastocysts. *Science* 1998; 282: 1145-7.
52. Reubinhoff BE, Pera MF, Fong CY, Trounson A, Bongso A. Embryonic stem cell lines from human blastocysts: somatic differentiation *in vitro*. *Nat Biotechnol* 2000; 18: 399-404.

Bone marrow-derived myogenic stem cells: a therapeutic alternative for muscular dystrophy?

Giulio Cossu[1], Fulvio Mavilio[2]

[1] Dipartimento di Istologia ed Embriologia Medica, Universita' di Roma "La Sapienza", Rome, Italy
[2] Gene Therapy Program, Istituto Scientifico H. San Raffaele, Milano, Italy

Cell and gene therapy for muscular dystrophy

Duchenne muscular dystrophy (DMD) is due to mutations in the dystrophin gene, encoding a component of the multi-protein complex linking the cytoskeleton of the muscle fiber to the extracellular matrix [1]. In the absence of dystrophin, the complex is functionally impaired, and the mechanical stress associated with contraction progressively leads to degeneration of the muscle fiber, wasting of skeletal muscle, progressive impairment of movements, and eventually paralysis and death [2]. In the first phases of the disease, new muscle fibers are formed by fusion of resident myoblasts, or satellite cells [3]. Once the proliferation potential of these cells is exhausted, the skeletal muscle is replaced by connective tissue [2].

The current therapeutic approaches to DMD involve pharmacological suppression of the inflammatory and immune responses, and achieve only temporary beneficial effects. More definitive, cell and gene therapy approaches range from injection of dystrophin-expressing adenoviral vectors (*in vivo* gene therapy) [4] to pharmacological up-regulation of the synthesis of the dystrophin-like protein utrophin [5, 6], to transplantation of allogeneic or autologous, genetically-modified myoblasts (*ex vivo* gene therapy). Each strategy has potential advantages and disadvantages, and none is ready to enter clinical practice at the moment. In particular, efficient delivery to diseased muscles of genetically-modified myoblasts, or even viral vectors carrying therapeutic genes, is one of the major hurdles currently limiting both *ex vivo* and *in vivo* approaches. Despite some anecdotal observations, it is generally accepted that satellite cells taken from skeletal muscle cannot colonize muscle tissue if delivered from the circulation. The availability of a cell population that could be engineered and then systemically delivered to a large number of muscles would therefore be essential for the development of a cell-mediated replacement therapy.

Myogenic progenitors from the bone marrow

Recently, we provided evidence that transplantable myogenic progenitors exist in the murine bone marrow, and that these cells may access the skeletal muscle *via* the peripheral circulation [7]. To identify these cells, we used a transgenic mouse line in which a *lacZ* gene encoding a nuclearly-targeted β-galactosidase is expressed under the control of muscle-specific regulatory elements (MLC3F-n*lacZ*). In these animals, the *lacZ* reporter is expressed only in striated muscle [8] and is therefore a sensitive marker of myogenic differentiation, both *in vitro* and *in vivo*. When cells from MLC3F-n*lacZ* mice are injected into regenerating muscle of immunodeficient mice, myogenic conversion is scored by the formation of muscle fibers with centrally-located, β-gal-positive nuclei. With this assay, we observed that unfractionated bone marrow gives rise to labeled muscle fibers with an unexpectedly high efficiency, suggesting the existence of progenitor cells endowed with myogenic potential in the bone marrow. To test whether these cells could be systemically delivered to the muscle, we transplanted MLC3F-n*lacZ* bone marrow into lethally-irradiated *scid/bg* mice, allowed the transplanted bone marrow to fully reconstitute the recipient animals, and then induced muscle regeneration by standard cardiotoxin injection into the *tibialis anterior* muscle. Histochemical analysis unequivocally showed the presence of β-gal-staining nuclei at the center and periphery of regenerated fibers, demonstrating for the first time that murine bone marrow contains transplantable progenitors that can be recruited to an injured muscle through the peripheral circulation, and participate in muscle repair by undergoing complete differentiation into mature muscle fibers [7]. If confirmed in humans, the existence of a transplantable cell that could be systemically delivered to a large fraction of muscles would open a new avenue in the development of a cell-mediated replacement therapy for muscular dystrophy [9].

The real therapeutic potential of such a strategy is, however, still questionable. Quantitatively, muscle repair by bone marrow-derived cells appeared in fact as a marginal phenomenon: in the muscles of the transplanted mice, less than 0.5% of the regenerated fibers contained β-gal-positive nuclei. On the other hand, a number of factors inherent to the experimental model were obviously limiting the overall efficiency of the system. First, bone marrow was transplanted in *toto* and according to a protocol optimized for hematopoietic stem cells. Under these conditions, not only the relative abundance of myogenic progenitors is unknown, but given the absence of any selective advantage, even their transplantation efficiency is difficult to determine. Second, resident myogenic precursors are perfectly healthy in *scid/bg* mice, and unaffected by the low-dose radiation administered before transplantation, and could therefore effectively compete with marrow-derived cells for muscle repair. As a matter of fact, our experiments indicated that marrow-derived progenitors have a slower differentiation kinetics compared to satellite cells, which respond faster to the regeneratory stimulus and, by the time marrow-derived cells come into the picture, have probably carried out much of the repair work. This kinetic difference might suggest that marrow-derived progenitors are recruited by the muscle injury but differentiate into more committed precursors rather than directly into muscle fibers, a hypothesis difficult to demonstrate since the MLC3F-n*lacZ* transgene is activated in differentiated fibers or in cells actively undergoing myogenic differentiation, but not in quiescent myoblasts [8]. This overall picture might substantially change in a dystrophic background, where a pool of normal or genetically-corrected cells could enjoy a selective advantage, and effectively replace a progressively exhausting pool of defective satellite cells.

In 1999, experiments carried out in Lou Kunkel's and Richard Mulligan's laboratory showed that dystrophin-deficient, *mdx* mice transplanted with the bone marrow of syngeneic C57BL/10 mice develop, eight to twelve weeks after transplantation, a small number of dystrophin-positive fibers containing genetically marked (Y chromosome) donor nuclei [10]. However, although the efficiency of muscle repopulation by marrow-derived progenitors appeared to be slightly higher in this model, the number of fibers carrying both dystrophin and the Y chromosome never exceeded 1% of the total fibers in the average muscle, showing that even in a chronically regenerating environment marrow-derived progenitors are unable to give rise to new muscle fibers in clinically relevant numbers. Similar experiments carried out in our laboratory in a slightly different animal model, the *mdx4cv* mutant characterized by an extremely low ($< 0.1\%$) background of revertant fibers, showed that the number of donor-derived, dystrophin-positive fibers does not increase with time, and never exceeds 0.5% of the total fibers as late as one year after bone marrow transplantation (unpublished observations).

From a clinical point of view, the studies on the *mdx* mice are a disappointment. They clearly indicate that either the number of myogenic progenitors present in a bone marrow transplant is insufficient to produce enough muscle mass, or that they are not transplanted as efficiently as the hematopoietic progenitors, or else that the *mdx* background does not provide enough selective advantage to these cells to trigger their expansion and ultimately a significant replacement of the resident satellite cell pool. In fact, one might argue that despite the dystrophin defect, the *mdx* mouse does not develop a dystrophic clinical phenotype (the musculature of these animals is actually hypertrophic), and that *mdx* satellite cells are perfectly capable of regenerating muscle for the entire animal's life span. The clinical picture is dramatically different in human muscular dystrophy, where the repair potential of muscle satellite cells is lost in the first years of a patient's life, and skeletal muscles undergo progressive and irreversible degeneration. In this situation, dystrophin-positive fibers made by transplanted bone marrow progenitors might have a selective advantage, resist degeneration, and progressively replace dystrophin-negative fibers. Care should therefore be exercised in extrapolating to humans the results obtained in *mdx* mice, while a different animal model is clearly needed to address any efficiency issue in a pre-clinical setting.

Multipotent stem cells: biological curiosity or new hope for cell transplantation?

In the course of their bone marrow transplantation studies, Gussoni *et al.* made the important observation that the muscle of C57Bl/10 mice contains a population of primitive cells (SP cells) which share the property of excluding a particular fluorescent dye (Hoechst 33342) with a sub-fraction of bone marrow containing primitive hematopoietic stem cells [11, 12]. Like bone marrow SP cells, muscle SP cells are capable of long-term hematopoietic reconstitution upon transplantation into *mdx* mice, and both give rise to dystrophin-positive muscle fibers eight to twelve weeks after transplantation [10]. Using a different technique, which involves some tissue culture steps, Margaret Goodell's group showed at the same time that the muscle tissue is a very abundant source of cells capable of long-term hematopoietic reconstitution in a serial transplantation assay, even more abundant than the bone marrow itself [13]. These data suggest, but do not prove, the existence of multipotent cells capable of differentiation into both the hematopoietic and the muscle cell lineage [14]. Multipotent stem cells may differentiate along alternative pathways depending on local cues provided by different tissue environments, or in response to specific recruitment signals. Are these discoveries providing grounds for an entirely new concept of cell therapy, based on transplantation of adult multipotent stem cells which can be induced to differentiate into specific tissues, or are they just showing a very remarkable property of a minor cell entity that we will never be able to use for practical purposes? A number of issues need to be addressed in order to provide an answer to this obviously crucial question.

First, do multipotent stem cells play a role in adult tissue homeostasis, or are they just a remnant of embryonic and fetal life which is rapidly lost after birth? Definitive hematopoietic stem cells derive from an earlier embryonic precursor with both angiogeneic and hematopoietic potential, which develops first in the embryonic aorta-gonad-mesonephros (AGM) region, and then migrates into the fetal liver, the spleen and eventually the bone marrow [15]. Giulio Cossu and his group have recently shown the existence of cells with muscle-forming capacity in the embryonic dorsal aorta [16]. *In vitro*, these cells express a number of myogenic and endothelial markers that are also expressed by satellite cells, including a receptor for vascular-endothelial growth factor (flk-1) VE-cadherin. *In vivo*, aorta-derived myogenic progenitors participate in muscle regeneration, and fuse with resident satellite cells [16]. These data suggest that a subset of post-natal myogenic cells may be rooted in a vascular lineage [17]. Whether these myogenic/vascular cells arise from a primordial pericyte, from endothelial cells proper, as suggested by the expression of endothelial markers, or from a circulating multipotent progenitor, is not currently known. Also unknown is the relationship, if any, of these cells with the primitive hemangioblast. The existence of self-renewing, multipotent hemato-angio-myogenic stem cells throughout embryonic, fetal and at least early post-natal life is suggested by the presence of myogenic progenitors in all hematopoietic tissues, *i.e.* dorsal aorta, AGM, fetal liver, and bone marrow ([16] and our unpublished observations). It is attractive to speculate that multipotent, hemato-angio-myogenic stem cells might colonize through the vasculature of developing tissues during embryogenesis, and adopt specific fates, such as satellite cells in the muscle or hematopoietic and mesenchymal stem cells in the bone marrow, depending on local environmental cues. If such "plastic" stem cells are preserved in the microvasculature of adult tissues, as the recent transplantation experiments would suggest, will we ever be able to identify, expand and transplant them in reasonable numbers? The absence of unique markers and the impossibility of carrying out clonal analysis in the only available assay of multipotentiality, transplantation *in vivo*, are at present clearly limiting our ability to better understand the biology of multipotent stem cell plasticity.

Second, can we induce expansion and differentiation of multipotent stem cells into a desired progeny *in vivo* at any reasonable efficiency? Analysis of the effect of cytokines and chemokines on the recruitment and differentiation of transplanted multipotent cells are just starting, and will hopefully provide new insight in the coming years. Recruitment and differentiation are clearly important factors to control in view of clinical application, since it is unlikely that we could re-create for non-hematopoietic tissues the selective ablation and competitive repopulation conditions that allowed bone marrow transplantation to become a clinical reality in the treatment of hematopoietic disorders.

Third, do multipotent stem cells exist in humans, and how can we assay for their abundance, plasticity, and clinical potential? These are really tough questions to answer, since *in vitro* assays thus far are unsatisfactory even for hematopoietic stem cells, and direct injection into immunodeficient mice might allow testing of the muscle-forming capacity of human cells isolated from the bone marrow, but not for their self-renewing capacity, plasticity, and recruitment through the peripheral circulation. Immunodeficient mouse strains that allow maintenance and expansion of very early human blood progenitors are available at the moment (*e.g.* the NOD/scid mouse), but do not allow complete differentiation into all the hematopoietic progenies, and are therefore unlikely to allow the analysis of even more complex phenomena such as recruitment and differentiation of a bone marrow-derived myogenic progenitor. More sophisticated human/mouse chimera are therefore to be developed for this specific purpose, while other pre-clinical models, such as non-human primates, need to be tested to get as close as possible to the human situation. Unfortunately, real models for human muscular dystrophy do not currently exist, or are very expensive (dystrophic dogs) and still very remotely related to the human situation. Given the still very primitive knowledge of the biology of marrow-derived myogenic progenitors, it is clearly too early to think about human clinical applications. Nevertheless, we should try do develop as soon as possible a consistent ethical framework to carry out future human trials, as well as a consensus as to what type of knowledge we should gain from the murine or from any other model before it becomes reasonable to start asking questions in a clinical setting.

The most attractive scenario for clinical application implies genetic modification and transplantation of autologous multipotent stem cells, a technology which has yet to be applied for the much better defined hematopoietic stem cell. The alternative is transplantation of normal, allogeneic cells. The treatments currently associated with clinical bone marrow transplantation involve radiation, and the use of toxic myeloablative drugs, and imply risks which should be seriously considered for non-cancer patients. Nevertheless, the lack of need for ablation of cancer cells might lead to the development of much milder protocols, which for fatal diseases like DMD might eventually become more than acceptable. It should also be considered that allogeneic bone marrow transplantation from a genetically normal donor could provide an additional but crucial benefit to dystrophic patients, that is, tolerization towards the dystrophin protein provided by the incoming, donor immune system. This could be an important factor, which might allow for the use of additional gene therapy in these patients without the risk of immune rejection of dystrophin-producing cells.

Stem cell biology is clearly coming of age, and raising new hopes that better fundamental knowledge and smart translational research might finally provide the tools for treating muscular dystrophy with cell and gene therapy. We will not have to wait too long to know whether this is just wishful thinking or an entirely new therapeutic perspective.

References

1. Nawrotzki R, Blake DJ, Davies KE. The genetic basis of neuromuscular disorders. *Trends Genet* 1996; 12: 294-8.
2. Emery A. *Duchenne muscular dystrophy*. Volume 1. New York: Oxford University Press, 1988.
3. Bischoff R. The satellite cell and muscle regeneration. In: Engel C, ed. *Myology, A. G. a. F.-A.* New York, N.Y.: McGraw-Hill, 1994.
4. Kochanek S, Clemens PR, Mitani K, Chen HH, Chan S, Caskey CT. A new adenoviral vector: Replacement of all viral coding sequences with 28 kb of DNA independently expressing both full-length dystrophin and beta-galactosidase. *Proc Natl Acad Sci USA* 1996; 93: 5731-6.
5. Deconinck N, Tinsley J, De Backer F, Fischer R, Kahn D, Phelps S, Davies K, Gillis JM. Expression of truncated utrophin leads to major functional improvements in dystrophin-deficient muscles of mice. *Nature Med* 1997; 3: 1216-21.
6. Tinsley JM, Potter AC, Phelps SR, Fisher R, Trickett JI, Davies KE. Amelioration of the dystrophic phenotype of mdx mice using a truncated utrophin transgene. *Nature* 1996; 384: 349-53.
7. Ferrari G, Cusella-De Angelis G, Coletta M, Paolucci E, Stornaiuolo A, Cossu G, Mavilio F. Muscle regeneration by bone marrow-derived myogenic progenitors. *Science* 1998; 279: 1528-30.
8. Kelly R, Alonso S, Tajbakhsh S, Cossu G, Buckingham M. Myosin light chain 3F regulatory sequences confer regionalized cardiac and skeletal muscle expression in transgenic mice. *J Cell Biol* 1995; 129: 383-96.
9. Partridge T. The "Fantastic Voyage" of muscle progenitor cells. *Nature Med* 1998; 4: 554-5.
10. Gussoni E, Soneoka Y, Strickland CD, Buzney EA, Khan MK, Flint AF, Kunkel LM, Mulligan RC. Dystrophin expression in the mdx mouse restored by stem cell transplantation. *Nature* 1999; 401: 390-4.
11. Goodell MA, Brose K, Paradis G, Conner AS, Mulligan RC. Isolation and functional properties of murine hematopoietic stem cells that are replicating *in vivo*. *J Exp Med* 1996; 183: 1797-806.
12. Goodell MA, Rosenzweig M, Kim H, Marks DF, DeMaria M, Paradis G, Grupp SA, Sieff CA, Mulligan RC, Johnson RP. Dye efflux studies suggest that hematopoietic stem cells expressing low or undetectable levels of CD34 antigen exist in multiple species. *Nature Med* 1997; 3: 1337-45.
13. Jackson KA, Mi T, Goodell MA. Hematopoietic potential of stem cells isolated from murine skeletal muscle. *Proc Natl Acad Sci USA* 1999; 96: 14482-6.
14. Lemischka I. The power of stem cells reconsidered? *Proc Natl Acad Sci USA* 1999; 96: 14193-5.
15. Dzierzak E, Medvinsky A, de Bruijn M. Qualitative and quantitative aspects of haematopoietic cell development in the mammalian embryo. *Immunol Today* 1998; 19: 228-36.
16. De Angelis L, Berghella L, Coletta M, Lattanzi L, Zanchi M, Cusella-De Angelis MG, Ponzetto C, Cossu G. Skeletal myogenic progenitors originating from embryonic dorsal aorta coexpress endothelial and myogenic markers and contribute to postnatal muscle growth and regeneration. *J Cell Biol* 1999; 147: 869-78.
17. Ordahl CP. Myogenic shape-shifters. *J Cell Biol* 1999; 147: 695-8.

Pluripotent Stem Cells: Therapeutic Perspectives and Ethical Issues
B. Dodet, M. Vicari, eds.
© John Libbey Eurotext, Paris, 2001

Ethical, legal and regulatory issues in the use of human embryonic stem cells in France

Claire Bonnat-Legras
Conseil d'État, Paris, France

The therapeutic prospects of stem cell research justify, according to the majority opinion, that the ban on embryo research written into French law in 1994 be revisited. First of all, I would like to briefly present the normative choices regarding the embryo and embryo experimentation which have been made in France in light of perspectives adopted in other countries and at the international level. On the basis of this underlying fabric, I will examine the ethical problems related to the utilisation of stem cells and, finally, outline the response that the Conseil d'Etat proposed to the Prime Minister in the November 1999 report on the revision of the French "Bioethics Laws".

The legal norms relevant to bioethics and the human embryo

Evolution of the debate regarding the embryo

This question symbolises the tensions and difficulties of the ethical debate raised by the development of life sciences. It may first be explained by the fact that the embryo poses in pure form the issue of respect for life from the moment it begins. With the development of a greater understanding of genetics, the embryo symbolises life for two reasons: the embryo is a carrier, from the first moments of its conception, of genetic characteristics of the person to be born, which belong to this person alone, in a world which attaches more and more importance to "genetic capital". As much by its potential for life as by the inherent fragility of what it materially is, that is to say, a mass of cells not even visible to the naked eye, the embryo represents, to quote Mrs. Neirinck [1], our humanity.

Until recently, the embryo did not pose a major problem to the French jurist; the Roman Law maxim of *infans conceptus* recognized the infant as a legal personality with property rights at birth. The debate on the legalisation of abortion, however, and the development of medically assisted procreation techniques have made the embryo the subject of intense philosophical, legal and political debates centred on two major questions: is the embryo a person from conception? What protection should it benefit from at different stages of its development?

The French position, today fixed by the January 17, 1975 law and by the July 1994 law, is based on of the following choices:

- **The French legislators did not find it necessary to give a definition of the human embryo or of the person.** They deemed that they should not or could not settle between the different philosophical options on the subject. However, they did say something about the embryo, since they defined the conditions which make the abortion or the creation and utilisation of an *in vitro* embryo are legal; they authorized its destruction as well, after a period of five years, if the embryo has not been claimed by the parents. The statute of the embryo, thus, is revealed in a certain way, *via* the limitations to the harm that can be done to them. We know that the embryo is not a person, otherwise the law of 1975 would legitimate homicide; nor is it a simple mass of cells, since it cannot be conceived *in vitro* except in the case of and according to the modalities of medically assisted procreation, under which the embryo may not be conceived for commercial ends and which includes a ban on all embryo experimentation.

The French legislators have neither made a choice regarding what the so called "human potentiality" – the embryo would be human on the condition that it would be recognized as such – nor that of progressive humanisation, confirmed only after the expiration of a certain delay or, for *in vitro* embryos, after implantation or gastrulation. The Parliament thus considered, following several scientists, that it was artificial to define the embryo by opposing it to the zygote or pre-embryo, which are concepts used in the United Kingdom and in Spain although they are perceived to be arbitrary. Science may have terms which designate the different stages of development of a human being, yet this does not necessarily result in a different representation of one's life and the respect it imposes as a function of the stage of development which is considered.

By refusing to develop a definition of the embryo or to create different legal regimes according to the different developmental stages, while defining rules applying to the embryo, the French Parliament has certainly paved the way for controversy. In fact, it is not unreasonable to think that *"it is the statute which must impose the limits, not the limits which impose the statute"* [2]. *"In 1975, he (the legislator) allowed for the destruction, but in 1994 allowed for the use of this embryo so difficult to define. So, have we here a legislator who speaks of what he cannot define? Or who declares himself selectively competent?"* [3]. The internal coherence of the law is in fact imperfect, notably, as is often remarked, where it prohibits experimentation on embryos while it authorizes their destruction.

By neither defining the person, nor the embryo, however, have not the legislators demonstrated a just understanding of their power? Giving the law the power, today, to qualify what a human being is in effect gives it the power to qualify otherwise tomorrow, in the worst case, to deny the personality of living beings. The person is stated and thus protected; the law needs go no further than to assure the protection due to each human being.

In most member States of the European Union, there is no legal definition of the human embryo (Belgium, Denmark, Finland, the Netherlands, Portugal, Sweden). Two countries have taken the opposite strategy: German legislation defines the embryo as *"a fertilised human ovule capable of developing, from fusion of the pronuclei"* while in British legislation, the embryo is understood as *"a living embryo resulting from completed fertilisation, including the ovule during fertilisation"*. Based on these relatively close definitions, these two countries have made opposite choices regarding experimentation on the embryo.

- **Second important point of the French bioethics norms: they logically trigger exceptions.** In 1975, the legislators began by stating the principle that the foetus can be considered as a human being; they then put this in the context of a logic of balancing this right with the consideration of situations where the mother is in distress and the danger that this presents, fixing the threshold of authorized abortion at up to ten weeks. Abortion was deliberately placed in the domain of transgression, in relation to this first definition.

The same structure is present in the 1994 law regarding medically assisted procreation and prenatal diagnosis. As in 1975, the French Parliament stated a position of principle but did not completely translate it into the law. Although article 2 of the July 29, 1994 law states that *"the law guarantees the protection of all human beings from the beginning of their life"*, the legislators did not make the choice to prohibit either the creation of supernumerary embryos or their frozen storage in anticipation of implantation in cases where previous attempts have failed. Article L. 152-8 of the Public Health Code, while considered to be very restrictive, also follows the idea of exceptions or balance: *"The* in vitro *conception of human embryos for research purposes is prohibited. All experimentation on the embryo is prohibited. With exceptional statute, the man and woman forming the couple may accept that studies be carried out on their embryos. These studies must have medical ends and not harm the embryo."*

Under very strict conditions, the embryo may thus be the subject of study and research with the aim of better understanding the mechanisms involved in its development and possible causes of miscarriage, particularly frequent in the human species. The July 29, 1994 law, however, clearly prohibits research on the *in vitro* embryo.

The choices relative to the ethical norm thus are amenable to critique: we may denounce, in the name of defence of the embryo, the problem of balance which determined these choices; we may also, like some editorials in the revue *Nature*, criticize this "ethic à la française" which deducts prohibitions from abstract principles, such as "the dignity of the human person" and which is dangerously paralysing research. France is actually closer to the deontological approach, which says that our duties and principles condition our actions and their consequences, it nevertheless makes a place for the utilitarian or teleological approach, which implies that human actions should be evaluated in function of the means taken and ends sought. The inspiration of the Bioethics Laws is thus impure for some, and balanced and reasonable for others.

It is true that, despite this critique, the laws of 1975 and 1994 have permitted, in a general way, both mediation of the debate and the moralisation of practices. The ethical norm must reflect a heightened standard, but it must also be respected: for this, it must navigate a balance between moral discipline and confidence in the freedom of the researcher, which drives him to search and find.

The international level

These principles, non-definition and the search for balance, have also inspired the more recent efforts which have resulted in the creation of international norms. At the European level, due to lack of consensus, no text concerning the embryo describes its statute in an explicit manner. The signatory countries of the Convention of the Council of Europe on Human Rights and Biomedicine, signed on March 4, 1997 in Oviedo, have not managed to agree on the legal statute of the embryo and therefore have not reached a decision concerning research on the embryo. They have thus sent this question back to the Member States, with the stipulation (article 18) that when research on embryos *in vitro* is permitted by the law, the law must assure adequate protection of the embryo; and the article continues by prohibiting the creation of human embryos for research purposes.

Following an amendment of the CDU by Edith Cresson, tending to prohibit the financing of embryo research at the Community level, the European group on Ethics in Science and New Technologies of the European Commission advocated, in an opinion on March 23, 1998, in the name of respect of the pluralism of ethical and legal approaches of the Member States, not to exclude Community financing for embryo researchers in countries where embryo experimentations is authorized, but with the condition that this financing be subject to strict legal and ethical conditions.

The Universal Declaration on Human Rights and the Human Genome adopted by UNESCO on November 11, 1997 does not take a position on the statute of the embryo.

Therapeutic prospects of stem cell research

Essentially, the ethical questions related to the utilisation of stem cells brings us back to a debate with well known terms culminating in the compromise described above. In fact, the development of medically assisted procreation techniques already posed the question of the nature of the *in vitro* embryo and noted the risk of its objectification, that is to say the danger that it would be considered as an object and, in the worst case, used as a material. The choice of balance, made in France, prohibited embryo research.

Reopening of the discussion regarding the ban on embryo research would be justified by the fact that the relevant research objectives have evolved: in 1994, embryo research aimed at finding ways to treat sterility or increasing the success rate of *in vitro* fertilisation by studying, notably, the benefit of certain culture conditions. The research which occupies the participants of this conference has a different objective. The majority here considers that the therapeutic perspectives of stem cell research should reopen the ethical debate. If stem cells are, as was affirmed before the Conseil d'Etat by scientists such as Yves Menezo, *"the therapeutic tool of the 3rd millennium"*, must a just balance between respect for life from its beginning and the right of those who suffer to see a collective undertaking of the most effective research to fight against their disease, be found? Are we considering two ethical principles of equal rank, which can be put in balance? In particular, is there a right of those who suffer that everything be done which might alleviate their suffering? A right of the gravely ill that medical research progresses, in a determined manner, to come to their aid? The comparison is not an easy one: on one side there is certain harm, on the other a potential interest, a simple therapeutic hope. We are thus before an ethical dilemma.

The prospects of regenerative medicine are in constant evolution and have again progressed since the Conseil d'Etat rendered its report last November. This situation asks for a concentrated effort on the part of scientists, lawyers and politicians to thoroughly understand the problems posed.

The ethical problems raised by stem cells are not homogenous. Certain techniques lead to the objectification of the embryo and, in any case, a modification of the balance developed by the French laws between the affirmation of the principle of protection and the recognition of targeted exceptions. Other techniques do not raise the same ethical objections.

The presentations that we have seen here have focused on two types of research:

1. The establishment of stem cell lines, capable of producing *in vitro* a great variety of cells and tissues, which opens exciting prospects for cell grafts and thus the treatment of diseases such as diabetes, leukaemia, multiple sclerosis, Parkinson's disease and Alzheimer's disease. Studies performed on rats presenting a myelinisation defect are a nice example[1]. This research may also be used to assure that a child not be a carrier of the same genetic defects as his parents or to better understand the developmental mechanisms of cancers.

2. Therapeutic cloning, eventually associated with transgenesis. Cloning by transfer of an adult nucleus or a nucleus from a blastocyst into an ovum allows for the creation of an embryo cultured *ex vivo*, the development of which will be stopped at a more or less precocious stage in order to obtain differentiated cells (heart, nerve, hematopoietic, etc.) for use in cell therapy. To solve histocompatibility problems, the production of ES cells by cloning based on ova reconstituted by nuclear transfer of somatic cells from the individual to be treated is envisioned; lines of immuno-compatible cells may be obtained that way.

Cloning also allows for the transgenic modification, *i.e.* by suppression or addition of a modified or intact gene, of the genetic characteristics of the *in vitro* embryo. First, a blastocyst generated by a couple carrying a genetic defect is used to obtain embryonic stem cells which will be corrected by transgenesis. Then, there are two possibilities: (i) microinjection of modified cells into an embryo at the morula or blastocyst stage, which will have little effect and which will not prevent that individual from transmitting the defect he carries; or (ii) the reconstitution of an embryo by introducing into the ovocyte of the woman of the couple the corrected nucleus of a cell derived from a blastocyst from the same couple. As explained by professor Thibault in an annex to the Conseil d'Etat's report, this second possibility is the only one which definitively eliminates the genetic defect while creating a reconstituted egg based on the genomes of the two parents. This genetic modification of nuclear donor cells implies the creation of a blastocyst.

The prospects of cellular therapy associated, or not associated, with cloning by nuclear transfer and transgenesis are thus exciting. At the same time, they raise notable ethical difficulties, which situate at two levels:

– **Which cells are involved?**

---

1. ES cells have been cultivated in the presence of two growth factors capable of provoking their differentiation into functional oligodendrocytes (characteristic morphology and myelin production). These cells, introduced into the spinal bone marrow and brain of a line of rats presenting a myelinisation defect analogous to Pelizaeus-Merzbacher's Disease (PBD), hereditary in humans, have multiplied, migrated from the site of injection and assured the myelinisation of 50% of the axons of these rats.

The use of cells from the internal cell mass of the blastocyst is obviously the target of the strongest objections. The utilisation of primordial germ cells (these cells, at the origin of reproductive cells of the testicle and ovary, are found in the posterior part of the embryo), which retain their pluripotency as long as they are not incorporated into the gonads and which can be recuperated following abortion, is acceptable, but subject to certain conditions to be defined which clearly differentiate the two acts; it can neither be considered as using the human being as an instrument, nor, I believe, as an act of "complicity" in abortion. However, professor Thibault explains that their potentiality is more limited than ES cells because their genome will not have undergone imprinting, the mechanism which renders either the male or female allele of a gene functional.

Remaining to be discussed are stem cells existing in adult organisms: recent research shows that the stem cells present in different types of tissue, where they foster renewal, are capable of behaving more or less as effectively as stem cells of other tissues. The research done with diabetic mice in Israel by Sarah Ferber's team, presented in the May 2000 issue of *Nature Medicine*, has also shown that pancreatic stem cells maintained in culture for three years continually produced islets of Langerhans; transplantation of these islets into diabetic mice restored a normal glucose level.

Embryonic cells derived from a blastocyst or primordial germinal cells appear, however, due to their pluripotency, the best models for understanding the process of cellular differentiation and serve as a basis for the elaboration of differentiated cell lines. It is in any case particularly important to assess whether the therapeutic resources anticipated from pluripotent stem cells present in the embryo during the first stage of development are much more considerable than those of somatic cells.

– **How will these cells be used?**

From the point of view of the French law, the therapeutic utilisation of stem cells is not acceptable if it leads to the objectification of the embryo. Under the May 27, 1997 Decree, which specifies the conditions for applying Article L. 152-8 of the Public Health Code, *in vitro* studies on the embryo must have medical ends and they must in no case harm the embryo. If the French legislators have thus not chosen the strictest respect of life from its beginning, they have in effect deemed that the use of an undeniably human being, whether for unselfish purposes or noble research aims, as a simple means is an affront to the dignity of the human being and represents an ontological bridge which they are not ready to cross.

In the name of this principle, it is not possible to permit the research necessary to develop the cell culture techniques since they do not respect the integrity of the embryo. Similar reasoning applies to the creation of cell lines developed from blastocysts, even when they are frozen and will not be used by the parent couple, thus leaving them only the option between "the trashcan and the microscope", as commented by Professor Sureau. Regarding the so-called "therapeutic cloning", this presupposes the creation of an *in vitro* embryo, the development of which will be terminated.

Must, as recommended by the French National Ethics Committee in their April 22, 1997 Opinion, reproductive cloning be distinguished from therapeutic cloning, the first being the sole reprehensible technique – as well as the sole technique prohibited by the additional protocol to the Oviedo Convention signed in Paris on January 12, 1998?

Does this distinction have a motivation other than obtaining a larger margin of acceptability for research?

Two justifications can be given for this distinction. The first focuses on the manner of obtaining the cloned embryos: according to some, like Henri Atlan [4], a mass of totipotent cells produced by nuclear transfer, without fertilisation, is not part of an embryo from the point of view of the manner in which it was produced. Its use, thus, cannot be considered as objectification of the embryo. But why then not say that an embryo produced *in vitro* is not the same thing as an embryo produced *in vivo*? A second type of justification is based on the ends of the cloning: it states that therapeutic cloning and reproductive cloning cannot be treated in the same manner because the motivation behind them is morally different: the first denies the identity and dignity of the human person while the second is inspired by the desire to prevent and heal serious diseases. This asks us to accept a moral doctrine which considers the ends of actions only, which does not convince me.

Considering transgenesis: beyond any reticence that one may have for therapeutic cloning, the definitive modification of genetic heritage of a human being is not an accepted notion.

On the ethical level, the principle of integrity of the human body mentioned by Article 16-4 of the French Civil Code prohibits any transformation of the genetic characteristic of a human person, *"without prejudice to research regarding the prevention and treatment of genetic disease"*. In other words, one exception to the principle of protection of the integrity of the genome is authorized by French law, with the aim of allowing for the prevention or treatment of genetic diseases. The text of the law itself, however, may prove to be an obstacle to treatment.

In the same vein, the European Council's January 25, 1999 decision determining the 1998-2002 life sciences research program excludes the support of activities destined to modify the genetic patrimony of individuals by hereditary alteration. The Oviedo convention also prohibits recourse to germ therapy; article 13 stipulates that an intervention aiming to modify the human genome should only be undertaken for preventative, diagnostic or therapeutic reasons and only if it does not aim to introduce a modification into the descendants genome.

Nevertheless, I believe that it should be recognised, as Professor Axel Kahn explained before the Conseil d'État, that germ-line therapy could be, in the future, the only way to correct certain serious genetic defects. We cannot follow those who affirm that, in the name of nature, we shouldn't modify the human being. That seems absurd to me: nature, as proclaimed by Sade, is most often confused with anti-nature. Above all, we are always changing nature; we don't let ourselves succumb in the presence of a serious disease. Still, added to ethical reticence is significant uncertainty regarding the possible consequences of germ-line therapy: certain scientists, such as Professor Jacques Montagut, point out that we do not know the ties that may exist between different sides of the genetic equation of each individual well enough to master the genetic reactions that would be required for germ-line therapy.

The proposition of the Conseil d'État

In the report on the revision of the bioethics laws submitted to the Prime Minister, the Conseil d'État pronounced itself in favour of the authorisation of research on the embryo *in vitro*, under the condition of strict regulation.

It esteemed that maintaining the prohibition on all research faced serious objections. *"A new point of equilibrium should be found between the respect of life since its very beginning which, in the strictest sense, leads to the prohibition of research on the embryo* in vitro *and the right of those with grave diseases to that which medical research, progressing in a determinant manner, can offer them."* In other words, it esteemed that these two imperatives were both essential ethical principles which had to be conciliated. Above and beyond ethical questions, other opportune elements and international comparison have influenced the ethical debate: in fact, the prohibition of embryo research in France has taken place within the context of its pursuit abroad. Thus, even if we refused to balance the principle of respect for life from its beginning and the question of delay for French research teams, we would still be left with the question of knowing if the prohibition on embryo research should permit the utilisation of embryonic cells cultivated abroad and, perhaps tomorrow, the prohibition of therapies based on such cells. It seems very difficult to respond positively without taking the risk of seeing such a position immediately stripped of effect by the departure of scientists, but also by "health tourism".

The Conseil d'Etat has thus proposed, in favour of the revision of the 1994 Bioethics Laws, a transition regime for authorisation of *in vitro* embryo research.

– Only two categories of embryos can be the object of research: embryos frozen *in vitro* which will not be used for a parental project and which will not be received by another couple and embryos produced *in vitro* and judged non-viable. That is to say, embryos which, by virtue of current legislation, may be destroyed. It is the progenators who, after having been specifically informed of the consequences of their decision, choose between the destruction of their embryos and their use in research.

The system chosen is an intermediary: the creation of embryos for research is prohibited, as well as the use of fresh embryos donated by a couple; on the contrary, the Conseil d'Etat could have chosen to allow research on those embryos created *in vitro* which are immediately destroyed because it is esteemed that they will not lead to the birth of a viable child: regarding these embryos, the research would have comprised, in fact, a scientific autopsy, which is already allowed.

– This research cannot result in the implantation of the concerned embryo. This is because research, by definition, has an experimental character which is incompatible with any acceptable risk concerning the child that would be born.

– This regime is proposed for a period of five years, particularly because it is recognised that science may lead to empty the debate of its contents, or at least calm its vivacity, with the development of technologies that provide pluripotent cells without the use of an embryo.

– Embryo research would be subject to case by case authorisation, by an agency created for this purpose.

– Finally, the Conseil d'État felt that the legislators decision not to define the embryo did not need to be revisited. It also refused to create a new category or to define a threshold below which experimentation would be authorised.

The Conseil d'Etat considered two questions

1. The risk that the prohibition on the production of embryos for research purposes will be bypassed. Will the creation of embryos be necessary to serve as a starting point for these theories? Or can these therapies be developed from orphaned frozen embryos?

2. An eventual slippery-slope effect: if we feel that opening research on embryos is justified for a single therapeutic end, it doesn't necessarily mean that we want to reverse the decision, made in 1994, to prohibit embryo research destined to ameliorate medically assisted procreation techniques, to develop new culture media, to improve methods of contraception and to understand gamete anomalies which, it seems, can be studied without fertilisation.

Conclusion

Is it more ethical to do all which is necessary to heal those with genetic diseases, or to respect the human being from the very beginning of life? Whatever answer to this question each one of us might have, I believe that it is essential that scientists, lawyers, politicians and the media are careful not to obscure the difficulties with terminological quarrels. It is an old French habit, a habit which is undoubtedly shared, to call something that serves our purpose by name and to call something that bothers us a problem: such is the "therapeutic" abortion, and "prevention" of Down's syndrome. In order for the ethical decision which will be made regarding embryo research to reflect, as best as possible, the convictions and morals of each citizen, the debate must be posed as purely as possible, without hiding behind language barriers erected for the needs of research. When the scientist speaks of the fertilised egg, the morula or the pre-embryo, he is referring to nothing other than the embryo in the common sense. When the National Consultative Ethics Committee speaks of therapeutic cloning, it doesn't help individuals themselves entirely grasp the ethical issues of this technique.

References

1. Neirinck. L'embryon humain ou la question en apparence sans réponse de la bioéthique. *Les petites affiches* n° 29, 9 mars 1998.
2. Baudoin JL, Labrusse-Riou C. *Produire l'homme: de quel droit?*, p. 205.
3. Memeteau G. La définition de la personne par la loi. *J Int Bioéthique* 1997: 39.
4. Atlan H et al. *Le clonage humain.* Paris: Le Seuil: 37.

# Ethical and biological aspects concerning the use of human embryonic stem cells and the legal situation in Germany

Gisela Badura-Lotter
Chair for Ethics in the Life Sciences, University of Tübingen, Germany

The first derivation and successful long term cultivation of human embryonic stem (ES) and germ (EG) cells in November 1998 [1, 2] was one of the most prominent scientific successes in the last few years. Science ranked it as the "breakthrough" of the year for 1999 [3]. Because of their theoretical potential to differentiate *in vitro* into every cell type of the body, human embryonic stem cells[1] are deemed to be very promising for many fields of medicine and biology. Researchers are especially interested in investigating their potential for transplantation medicine. Knowledge from animal experiments seems to encourage the idea of cell and tissue therapies based on the use of embryonic stem cells [4]. However, only a few experiments with animals addressing the derivation, purification and long-term behaviour of transplanted differentiated cells have been carried out so far and only one study especially addressing the *in vitro* differentiation capacity of human embryonic stem cells has been published so far [5]. Given the potential of embryonic stem cells to develop into teratomas (for which it is necessary to have 100% pure colonies of differentiated cells prior to transplantation trials), the yet unfulfilled demand for stable integration and physiological functioning of the transplanted cells, and the as yet unsolved immunological problems which exist, it seems premature to promise a revolution in transplantation medicine. Although ideas to overcome immune rejection, especially with the aid of genetically modified embryonic stem cells, comprise one of the most exciting perspectives in this new field of scientific research, there is at present no evidence that the envisioned strategies will work. There is a great demand for further studies on animal models, such as mouse and rat, which must be done before one could take the responsibility for recommending the use of human embryonic stem cells in clinical trials.

But perhaps there are other less spectacular but nevertheless perhaps not less promising research fields for human embryonic stem cells. The use of embryonic stem cells from animals in drug testing and toxicology has been investigated quite successfully in recent years [6-8]. It seems likely that *in vitro* differentiated human embryonic stem cells could be used for the same purpose. It might then be possible to test the effects of drugs and unknown agents on specific cells and tissues and, most of all, reliable

---

1. I will use the expression embryonic stem cells and embryonic germ, for both ES or EG cells. When it is necessary to distinguish between the two, I will use the word ES cells or EG cells.

methods to test embryotoxic effects might then evolve. A reduction in the use of animals in pharmacological and toxicological tests might be a possible, desirable side effect.

Another field of scientific interest lies in the use of human embryonic stem cells in fundamental biological research on molecular embryology. These cells might offer new ways to investigate genetic and biochemical mechanisms in early human development *in vitro*.

The fourth envisioned application for human embryonic stem cells is the above mentioned gene therapy. The idea is to first modify an enucleated human egg by transfer of a somatic nucleus from the prospective recipient with the aim of overcoming immune rejection. This egg would then be allowed to develop to the blastocyst stage, at which point the ICM (inner cell mass) would be removed and ES cells cultured. The ES cells could then be additionally modified using homologue recombination techniques to introduce specific DNA segments. These modified ES cells could then be differentiated *in vitro* to the desired cell type – equipped with the additional "therapeutic" DNA and transplanted in the recipient without any rejection. Science fiction? It seems possible and even realistic enough for the Geron Corporation to have engaged in the nuclear transfer strategy by fusing with the Roslin Biomed ("Dolly") last year for the explicit purpose of using it in combination with ES cells. However, these options are in the very basic stage of theoretical consideration – at least as far as is publicly known.

That is the gist of aims of research on embryonic stem cells. I hope it has become clear that knowledge about human embryonic stem cells is very limited. All we know is based on only three publications and animal experimentation, which is surely only in part helpful and applicable to human beings. Some scientists plead for a careful assessment of this technique – especially in the light of the more or less disappointing outcome of the formerly glorified gene therapy. On the other hand, some researchers claim that the use of embryonic stem cells is the only way to facilitate large scale cell and tissue therapies (especially in neuro-degenerative and heart diseases) regardless of our limited knowledge. Such statements neglect the rapid and formerly unexpected developments in somatic stem cell research. It has recently been shown that the developmental capacity of neural stem cells is broader than previously assumed [9]. Clarke *et al.* demonstrated that neural stem cells from the adult mouse brain can contribute to the formation of chimeric chick and mouse embryos and give rise to cells of all germ layers. It may be possible to simulate *in vitro* the factors influencing the diverse differentiation of neural stem cells *in vivo*. Such a model could then be used for the same purposes as embryonic stem cells but without the use of human embryos or foetuses.

Of course these first findings are only a promising foundation for further research and not the ultimate path to be taken by transplantation medicine. However, it might help to remember that the field of stem cell research is wide and that the public focus on embryonic stem cells seems somewhat excessive. This great public concern might partly be due to the reactions of the scientific community which, as I already mentioned, celebrated the first derivation of human embryonic stem cells in 1998 as one of science's major steps. But I think the "omnipresence" of the topic in the media has also been due to the legal and ethical debate that started one year earlier after the 13th International Congress of Developmental Biology in Snowbird, at which John Gearhart shared his vision of the cultivation of human embryonic germ cells by the scientists of his laboratory.

The legal situation in Germany

I would now like to go into the legal situation in Germany, and in doing so explain why I have put so much emphasis on the description of the "state of the art" in embryonic stem cell research. It is because research involving human embryonic and foetal material is the subject of legal and ethical restrictions in most countries. It is a widely shared consensus, especially in European countries, that human embryos and foetuses have at least some sort of moral status that protects them from being uncontrollably used for the purpose of others. That means that where research on human embryos is allowed, *e.g.* in Great Britain, it is restricted to specific research purposes which must be accepted by a Commission. As I will argue below, it is not self-evident that research on human ES cells can meet sufficient criteria to outweigh the destruction of early human life, especially with regard to the possible alternative options.

In Germany, which has one of the most restrictive laws on embryo research in Europe[2], research on human embryos is prohibited by criminal law. The protected subjects of the law are the embryo as defined below and the woman undergoing *in vitro* fertilisation who will carry the embryo. An embryo – as defined by the German Embryo Protection Act – is: *"the fertilised human egg, capable of development, from the moment of the fusion of the cell nuclei, and further every totipotent cell extracted from an embryo, which is capable of dividing and developing into an individual if the necessary conditions are provided"*[3]. The German Embryo Protection Act prohibits every *in vitro* experiment with a human embryo which does not pursue the well-being of the embryo. Therefore the derivation of human ES cells is prohibited in Germany. This is not the case concerning the derivation of human EG cells, because the use of aborted foetuses does not fall under the Embryo Protection Act and is also not prohibited elsewhere[4]. The use of dead foetuses is subject to the guidelines for the use of foetal cells and foetal tissues of the Bundesärztekammer, which is the head organisation of German physicians. The guidelines allow the extraction of cells for scientific, therapeutic and diagnostic purposes under certain conditions.

It is not certain, however, whether ES cells can be imported from other countries like the United States or Great Britain, where the use of embryos for research purposes is permitted. Import of ES cells would be legal (under certain restrictions) on the condition that they are pluripotent, because the use of totipotent cells (as mentioned above) is prohibited. It would be allowed because the general principle employed is the principle of territoriality, the *lex loci*, provided for in § 3 of the Criminal Code which connects the culpability of a person with the state where the crime was committed. It would therefore be legal for a German scientist to buy ES cells from a company which already provides the cell lines commercially. A German scientist would not be allowed to commission someone to derive ES cells in another country, *e.g.* the United States. He

---

2. Only in Austria is legislation comparably strict.
3. Original text: *"Als Embryo im Sinne dieses Gesetzes gilt bereits die befruchtete, entwicklungsfähige menschliche Eizelle vom Zeitpunkt der Kernverschmelzung an, ferner jede einem Embryo entnommene totipotente Zelle, die sich bei Vorliegen der dafür erforderlichen weiteren Voraussetzungen zu teilen und zu einem Individuum zu entwickeln vermag."* In Keller/Günther/Kaiser, 1992. English translation by the author.
4. For further detail see [10].

must also not pay another scientist to do the work (*i.e.* in this case: destroying an embryo to extract the inner cell mass) in another country.

Due to these difficulties concerning the legal situation in Germany, some scientists call for reducing the restrictions or even want to repeal the Embryo Protection Act. They found their arguments on the enormous potential for science and medicine that would be provided by human ES cells and the claim sometimes made that no adequate alternatives are available. However – as argued above –, research on human embryonic stem cells is not applied research but rather basic research, at least as long as it is conducted in a responsible way. Furthermore, there are alternative research options, not only for the main medical purpose of cell and tissue therapy but at least for pharmacology and toxicology as well. We don't know substantially more about the feasibility of those alternative options, *i.e.* somatic or cord blood stem cells, tissue engineering or new artificial organs, than we know about the feasibility of successful cell therapies based on the use of human embryonic stem cells. Therefore the far reaching promises made by some researchers are, in my opinion, not good scientific practise. The decision, as to whether to allow or to facilitate research on human embryos must be made through a democratic process, at least in democratic countries. We as scientists who are involved in this decision-making process have the duty to inform the political decision makers as comprehensively and honestly as possible.

The ethical debate

The ethical debate has been somehow focused on the ethical problem of the moral status of the human embryo and foetus, since the derivation of human ES and EG cells is not possible without the destruction of an early human embryo or of an aborted embryo/foetus, respectively. The key point for the decision whether embryo research is ethically acceptable or not seems to lie in the question concerning the moral status of the entities concerned. But regarding the long history of the "embryo debate", it must be stated that no convincing basic theory that would give a universally acceptable foundation of the moral status of the human embryo has been developed so far. In contrast, different views about the moral status of early human life has been established in different theories, in European laws, the European public and the scientific community. Some researchers hold the view that they are only following the usual scientific process when they claim to work with human embryonic stem cells, *i.e.* to pursue all the different pathways available in stem cell research to find out if one will work out or which of them shows to be the most promising. They don't see an "intuitive barrier" in using human blastocysts for the derivation of stem cells. But many of those researchers do have ethical problems with the idea of manipulating human embryos, with the implicit possibility of a transfer into a woman's uterus, or the germ line. On the other hand, there is a community of scientists and physicians who would – intuitively or due to their moral convictions – not work on human embryos but rather prefer to follow alternative routes of stem cell research.

Having ascertained the pluralistic treatment of that problem in the different parts of our societies so far, the question which now arises is whether the ethicists have to capitulate in light of what could be described in a negative sense as a form of ethical relativism. I think not. An answer might be found by departing from the narrow pathway of either the "moral status debate" or on the other hand the "practical compromise solution" of allowing the carefully controlled use of human embryos only for the derivation of stem cells (as it is discussed in Germany). The first only offers a narrow perspective of the vast field of embryo research and its manifold meanings for our societies. The second does not solve the ethical problem and is in all probability not even practical because legislation, especially in Germany, cannot limit embryo research to a single specific field.

Given the assumptions that: (1) research on human ES cells does require the destruction of human embryos and (2) a legal restriction of embryo research to the derivation of ES cells is not feasible, we can ask the question: "Do we principally want to allow research on human embryos or not[5]?"

At this point, I might have to grasp upon a frequently used argument which states that only a limited number of blastocysts would have to be used even to meet the demands of widespread research activities because of the capacity of ES cells to proliferate in their undifferentiated state indefinitely *in vitro*. This is undoubtedly true. But, as the latest debate in Great Britain about a possible approval of cloning shows[6], the most favoured conception of how to overcome immune rejection (*i.e.* to put a recipient's somatic cell nucleus into an enucleated egg, as described above) would require at least one embryo for each transplantation patient. And this is only true on the assumption that the technique will be developed to the point where one would not need – as in the "Dolly trials" – more than 200 eggs for one successful transfer not counting the embryos which would be used to promote the technique to that point.

So if we admit that a moderate use of human embryos is acceptable for the aim of developing cell and tissue transplantation therapies, we have to state that the most elegant way to reach that aim is not acceptable. So one should at least promote other strategies for overcoming immune rejection like establishing ES cell banks with all major HLA types or reprogramming of the recipient's somatic cell directly to a pluripotent stem cell stage.

However this would still involve a considerable exploitation of human embryos and we would still be asked to decide whether we as a society want that or not. I cannot at this point draw a whole sketch of an ethical theory that would address the question in the way I think it could reasonably be done. I just want to raise some questions that are still to be answered and that might help to develop a more comprehensive picture of the situation.

Besides the medical problems mentioned above, there are some aspects concerning the individual as well as society as a whole. Research on human embryos involves the acquisition of embryos. If the demand exceeds the supply, which is at the moment constituted by the so-called "spare embryos" provided by clinics offering *in vitro* fertilisation, would it be acceptable to create human embryos for research purposes? Or

---

5. I would like to follow a distinction made by Hans Kämer in 1992 [11]. He showed that for a practical philosophy it is necessary to distinguish between a strong "moral philosophy" (represented in the question: what do I/we have to do?) and a modern "Strebensethik" (represented in the question what do I/we want to do, *i.e.* how do I/we want to live a good life?). In the context of embryo research I leave the field of "moral philosophy" for the above mentioned reasons and think it is more helpful to address the ethical problem from a "strebensethische" point of view.
6. BBC News, Monday 3 April: "UK to 'approve therapeutic cloning'". http://news.bbc.uk Sci/Tech.

would it alter the practise of hormonal stimulation during *in vitro* fertilisation trials? Would the use of dead foetuses alter the practise of abortion? To ask these questions from another point of view: could it be guaranteed that a wide use of embryonic stem cells in transplantation medicine and pharmacology would not lead to a "source shortage"? I think it is necessary to follow the whole course of possible scenarios and to reflect about solutions to potential problems before they can impose a "normative pressure".

Furthermore, there are critical voices which connect the question of embryo research to the one of common human rights. If we allow research on early human embryos because they do not display the characteristics of human persons, *i.e.* self-consciousness and rationality, we start to make human rights dependent on specific characteristics and not on the human genus as such. It might erode the idea of human rights principally, if we accept such a division of human life. I think it is hardly possible to assess such "slippery slope" arguments in a way as to predict their probability. But it might be worth considering their implications.

Knowing that there are far more aspects to consider, I would like to draw your attention to a last point, which I call a biographical argument. I think we can state that a person experiences his or her life as a continuous process and his- or herself as a continuous, though changing, individual from the beginning of development. I want to raise the question as to whether it would be a violation of human (and personal) integrity if a certain phase of development is excluded from protection by human rights. If in this phase of development serious genetic or other biological manipulations of the body, as well as its use for the interests of others and even the destruction of someone's life is possible, wouldn't that alter our self understanding dramatically? Just to know that it was to the legitimate decision of others not to be killed during a certain phase of one's life must alter the understanding of our own life, which is so far constituted by the strong feeling that we have the right to absence of bodily harm the whole life long, even if we are not actually able to claim this right. I am sure that there will be different opinions about the significance of such an impact. But I would like you to consider that embryo research is not an isolated scientific field. It is and will be connected to other areas like *in vitro* fertilisation techniques, preimplantation diagnoses and therapies, somatic and germline gene therapy and others. The availability of the human embryo will create more ways of defining and constructing the physical (and emotional) constitution of a person. Human freedom, which is the constitutional basis for our capacity for responsibility, will diminish to the extent that the contingency of our "so-being" lies in the responsibility of others.

References

1. Thomson JA *et al.* Embryonic stem cells lines derived from human blastocysts. *Science* 1998; 282: 1145-7.
2. Shamblott MJ *et al.* Derivation of pluripotent stem cells from cultured human primordial germ cells. *Proc Natl Acad Sci USA* 1998; 95: 13726-31.
3. Vogel G. Breakthrough of the year: capturing the promise of youth. *Science* 1999; 286: 2238-9.
4. Brüstle O *et al.* Embryonic stem cell-derived glial precursors: a source of myelinating transplants. *Science* 1999; 285: 754-6.

5. Reubinoff BE *et al.* Embryonic stem cell lines from human blastocysts: somatic differentiation *in vitro*. *Nat Biotechn* 2000; 18: 399-404.
6. Guan K *et al.* Embryonic stem cells *in vitro* – prospects for cell and developmental biology, embryotoxicology and cell therapy. ALTEX, Vol. 16, 1999: 135-41.
7. Scholz G *et al.* Ergebnisse der ersten Phase des ECVAM-Projektes zur Prävalidierung von drei *in vitro* Embryotoxizitätstests. ALTEX, Vol. 15, 1998: 3-8.
8. Spielmann H *et al.* The embryonic stem cell test, an *in vitro* embryotoxicity test using two permanent mouse cell lines: 3T3 fibroblasts and embryonic stem cells. *Vitro Toxicol* 1997; 10: 119-27.
9. Clarke DL *et al.* Generalized potential of adult neural stem cells. *Science* 2000; 288: 1660-3.
10. Wolfrum R, Zeller AC. Legal aspects of research with human pluripotent stem cells in Germany. *Biomed Ethics* 1999; 4: S. 102-7.
11. Krämer H. *Integrative Ethik*. Frankfurt a.M.: Suhrkamp Taschenbuch Verlag, 1991.

Pluripotent Stem Cells: Therapeutic Perspectives and Ethical Issues
B. Dodet, M. Vicari, eds.
© John Libbey Eurotext, Paris, 2001

Ethical, legal and regulatory issues in the use of human embryonic stem cells in the United Kingdom

Sheila A.M. McLean
Institute of Law and Ethics in Medicine, University of Glasgow, Scotland, United Kingdom

Unlike some of its European colleagues, the United Kingdom arguably has a relatively relaxed attitude towards the use of embryos and embryonic material for research purposes. The Human Fertilisation and Embryology Act 1990 permits the creation of embryos for research purposes [1] and the use of donated embryos. However, this is not a completely unfettered authority to engage in embryo research. Schedule 2 of the legislation states that research can only be licensed if the Human Fertilisation and Embryology Authority (HFEA) believes it to be necessary or desirable for one of the following purposes:

– promoting advances in the treatment of infertility,

– increasing knowledge about the causes of congenital disease,

– increasing knowledge about the causes of miscarriage,

– developing more effective techniques of contraception, or

– developing methods for detecting the presence of gene or chromosome abnormalities in embryos before implantation,

– or such other purposes as may be specified in regulations by the Secretary of State [2].

The legislation covers research on any embryo which is created *ex vivo*, and any licensed research can take place only within the first 14 days of the existence of the embryo [3][1].

Despite the fact that this is now settled law, objections to the creation and use of embryos for these purposes continue. Objections, which might broadly be described as ethical, can take two forms. First, it may be argued that the embryo of the human species is entitled to respect – a respect which should preclude their creation for, or use in, research projects. Unsurprisingly, proponents of this view would generally also be anti-abortion. From their perspective, it is wrong to treat a human embryo as if it

---

1. See also [4], noting that *"the following activities are prohibited by law: a) keeping or using an embryo after the appearance of the primitive streak or after 14 days, whichever is the earlier...".* These guidelines were updated in 1998. A full text can be found at the HFEA website http://www.hfea.gov.uk.

were a means to an end, and wrong to deliberately inflict potential harm on it, including denying it the opportunity of implantation after creation (which is mandatory in terms of the legislation) [4], [5][2], [6][3].

A second form of objection, which does not depend on the first, although it may co-exist with it, could be taken to the type of research which it is intended to perform. This objection would concede that some research is morally permissible, but would argue that the type of research is critical to its morality. Given that the first objection was not deemed sufficient by United Kingdom law makers, they concerned themselves ultimately with the second form of objection. It was in response to this that the HFE Act was specific about the purposes for which embryos may be used – generally speaking sticking to research projects which were thought to have a "good" outcome – and specifically sought to outlaw cloning, a technique which has been universally condemned.

Next generation research

However, although the HFE Act is now apparently widely accepted, it was promulgated at a time when the science of stem cell research was in its infancy, and certainly its potential use in humans was a long way in the future. For this reason, the Act is essentially silent on this matter. In certain situations, of course, stem cell research may involve the creation of an *in vitro* embryo, and the Act would therefore apply. In others, there is a real possibility that cloning technology will need to be used; here the Act might be thought to be clear. However, the terms of the legislation expressly outlaw a particular form of cloning, namely *"... replacing a nucleus of a cell of an embryo with a nucleus taken from the cell of another person, another embryo, or a subsequent development of an embryo"* [7] and do not in reality preclude all possible cloning techniques. Nonetheless, the Government and the HFEA are apparently comfortable that their existing powers would be sufficient to ensure that any project which could lead to human cloning, in whatever form the technology takes, would not be licensed in the United Kingdom [8].

It is not the purpose of this chapter to consider in any depth the kinds of research which might in the future prove possible. Rather, the text will seek to evaluate some of the ethical and legal arguments surrounding stem cell research, particularly in light of the recent publication by the Nuffield Council of its Report "Stem Cell Therapy: The Ethical Issues" [8]. Subsequent to the publication of the Nuffield Council's Report, the Government's Chief Medical Officer issued a Report in June, 2000, which essentially agreed with the proposition that stem cell research should be permitted [9]. Their recommendations will be considered as part of what follows. Significantly, both the Nuffield Report, and the CMO's Report challenge the recent Government rejection of a joint report by the Human Genetics Advisory Commission and the Human Fertilisation and Embryology Authority [10]. This report, using a distinction between repro-

---

2. *"... embryos which have themselves been subject to procedures which carry an actual or reasonable theoretical risk of harm to their development potential should not be used for treatment"* [5].
3. Further, the Code of Practice says: *"embryos which have been appropriated for a research project must not be used for any other purposes"* (original emphasis).

ductive and therapeutic cloning, had argued that the terms of the 1990 Act should be extended to include:

- developing methods of therapy for mitochondrial diseases,
- developing methods of therapy for diseased or damaged tissues or organs.

Interestingly, the Government has signalled its lack of objection to the CMO's Report, which will be debated in Parliament in the future. An open vote will be allowed.

The Nuffield Report

The Report tackles head on the kinds of arguments there may be against permitting stem cell research to develop. It has already been noted that one possible objection to the use of embryos for research is that – no matter the aim of the research – it is disrespectful to the embryo. On this point, the Report concludes:

"A donated embryo has been created with a view to implantation in the uterus. Once it is not implanted, it no longer has a future and, in the normal course of events, it will be allowed to perish or be donated for research. We consider that the removal and cultivation of cells from such an embryo does not indicate a lack of respect for the embryo. Indeed, such a process could be regarded as being analogous to tissue donation [11]."

The CMO's Report, also addressed this issue, and concluded as follows:

"It is not possible to reconcile the opposing views on the moral status of the embryo and on the use of embryos in research. There are those for whom any use of an embryo in such research is morally objectionable and cannot be balanced by the potential benefits. However, those with such a view must be opposed to all research on embryos, not just to these new uses. The Expert Group accepted the 'balancing' approach which commended itself to the majority of the Warnock Committee. On this basis, extending the permitted research uses of embryos appears not to raise new issues of principle [12]."

Thus, in their conclusion, there is no disrespect to such an embryo by using it as part of a research project. Equally, they note that the potentially more thorny question of deliberately creating embryos for such research is not one which currently needs to be tackled as there would appear to be a sufficiency of donated embryos [13][4].

The second argument against using embryos, referred to earlier, relates to the *kind* of research which is undertaken. Although we might concede that *some* research is permissible, it might nonetheless appear that boundaries should be drawn. Thus, arguably, while it is permissible to use embryos in the ways described in the legislation, it

---

4. *"As long as there are sufficient and appropriate donated embryos from IVF treatments for use in research, the Council takes the view that there are no compelling reasons to allow additional embryos to be created merely to increase the number of embryos available for ES cell research or therapy. However, we suggest that this issue be kept under review"* [13].

might be thought a step too far to extend the legitimate uses of embryos. However, in the Nuffield Council's view, *"... there are no grounds for making a moral distinction between research into diagnostic methods or reproduction which is permitted under UK legislation and research into potential therapies which is not permitted"* [13]. As has already been seen, this view was also taken by the CMO's Report.

In a passage which clearly explains the Nuffield Council's arguably pragmatic approach to the use of human embryos, their position on the general principle of using embryos as a means to an end is clarified:

"Research into potential therapies is not qualitatively different from research into diagnostic methods of reproduction. Neither benefits the embryo upon which research is conducted, but both may be of benefit to people in the future. Each form of research involves using the embryo as a means to an end but, since we accept the morality of doing so in relation to currently authorised embryo research, there seems to be no good reason to disallow research on the embryo where the aim of the research is to develop therapies for others [14]*."*

From their perspective, then, the ethical arguments do not stand up to scrutiny. It must, of course, be noted that this is only a tenable position if we agree on two things. First, it must be accepted that research on human embryos is *in itself* ethical. Clearly, those who continue to oppose the terms of the HFE Act will be unconvinced by the Nuffield Council's arguments, which are essentially second-order. For opponents, the fact that something "bad" is being done already would be no justification for adding to it. Arguably, therefore, the Nuffield Council's Report will do little if anything to satisfy this group. Having said that, there is a certain resonance in its conclusions which would be likely to convince those who have no fundamental objection to the use of human embryos as research subjects.

Second, of course, in order to support the Nuffield Council's view that the 1990 legislation should be amended specifically to include research *"... for the purpose of developing tissues to treat diseases from derived embryonic (ES) cells..."* [13], and, by analogy research into SCNT and other *"forms of reprogramming the nuclei of human somatic cells"* [13] where such research falls to be licensed by the HFEA, it may be necessary to be satisfied that the second ethical objection outlined above can be met. Thus, it may be that we would need to be satisfied that the type of research envisaged i) was not in some way disregarding the respect due to the embryo and ii) would result in some good. It is here that some doubts about the reasoning of the Nuffield Council can be expressed.

Clearly the Nuffield Report's conclusions were heavily influenced by what its authors evidently saw as the enormous potential of stem cell research. Although they acknowledge the problems or difficulties which may be associated with it, they conclude that, *"the potential scope of this technology and the range of its applications are very wide"* [15]. In addition, they continue:

"Recent research suggests that human stem cells can give rise to many different types of cells, such as muscle cells, nerve cells, heart cells, blood cells and others. They raise

the possibility, therefore, of major advances in healthcare... The availability of stem cells may also change the way that drugs are tested. New drugs could be tested for safety and efficacy on cultured liver or skin cells derived from stem cells before being tested on humans. Further research on stem cells also promises to improve our understanding of the complexities of normal human development [16]."

However, there must be some doubt about the extent to which we can be entirely sanguine about the use of human embryos for these purposes. Other papers in this collection will show just how far away we are from realistically reaping any of the potential benefits of stem cell research. Indeed, it might be argued that this technique may be overtaken by alternative methods of meeting the therapeutic needs which it is designed to meet. If either of these considerations is valid, then there is a legitimate question about whether or not the arguments in favour of permitting research in this area fall at the hurdle of the second ethical objection. In addition, the CMO's Report expressly concedes that the potential good that may come from this research is a long way off. As the Report says, *"most of the scientists in this field see many technical and scientific hurdles to be overcome before the potential benefits of stem cell techniques could be realised"* [17].

Nonetheless, given the approach adopted by the Nuffield Council, the ground was prepared to explore the way forward. As has already been noted, the joint report from HGAC and HFEA received a cool reception from Government. This was almost certainly based on the public concern about the possibility of cloning technologies being used for reproductive purposes. However, at least one form of cloning is specifically outlawed in the UK, and, as we have seen, there seems reason to believe that other techniques which are not specifically referred to in the Act would also be covered by the regulatory framework of the legislation. In any event, the joint report at no stage suggested that reproductive cloning should be permitted. Rather, it concentrated on therapeutic cloning – that is, for example, the use of cloning technologies to generate replacement tissue and organs.

Manifestly, it is this area in which cutting edge research is most likely to make an impression – albeit that this seems still to be a long way off.

Consent

Unsurprisingly, one of the major concerns in this area relates to the question of consent. Under Schedule 3 of the HFE Act, individuals must specify the uses which can be made of embryos derived from their gametes. This must follow the opportunity for counselling and the adequate provision of information. The creation of ES cell lines is, however, seen to be different from the research currently permitted in the legislation. Where cell lines are developed, and although the embryo will require to be destroyed post research, the DNA of the donating couple will live on in the cell line. Theoretically, therefore it may be possible to trace the cell line back to the genetic donors. This, the Nuffield Council believes, requires that specific consent should be required before embryos can be used in this way [18]. If this is to be done, it would meet the general intention of the 1990 Act, and presumably, given the sensitivity of the activity, consent would be required in writing[5], potentially requiring minimal legislative amendment.

Although it has been suggested that the Nuffield Report could be seen by some as somewhat cavalier in its approach to the use of embryos for stem cell research, it is by no means unaware of the sensitivities involved. In respect of consent, the Report specifically endorses the recommendations of the US National Bioethics Advisory Commission Report (1999) [21] that:

"During the presentation about potential research use of embryos... the person seeking the donation should:

– disclose that the ES cell research is not intended to provide medical benefit to embryo donors;

– make clear that consenting or refusing to donate embryos to research will not affect the quality of any future care provided to prospective donors;

– describe the general area of the research to be carried out with the embryos and the specific research protocol, if known;

– disclose the source of funding and expected commercial benefits of the research with the embryos, if known;

– make clear that embryos used in research will not be transferred to any woman's uterus, and

– make clear that the research will involve the destruction of the embryos."

Researchers may not promise donors that ES cells derived from their embryos will be used to treat patient-subjects specified by the donors [21].

Embryonic germ cells

Finally, the Nuffield Report turns its attention to the derivation of embryonic germ cells. They note that this too is a controversial area, not least because it is tied to the ethical acceptability of abortion. Once again, for those who are unalterably opposed to abortion, the "sin" is effectively compounded by using the embryo (or foetus) in this way. However, the Nuffield Report notes that cadaveric foetal tissue is already used in this way, and that research ethics committees have already approved the use of cadaveric foetal tissue in the treatment of Parkinson's disease [22].

There would, therefore, be no specific reason why embryonic tissue derived from abortion could not be used in the same way. Interestingly, this would not be covered by the HFE Act (which only covers embryos created *in vitro*) and would be subject therefore only to the scrutiny of research ethics committees, and any available guidelines (and of course the terms of the Abortion Act 1967 (as amended). Again the Nuffield Council sees great advantages in using EG cells, specifically in relation to the creation of cell lines for transplantation.

---

5. For a discussion of the written consent provisions of the legislation, see [19] and [20].

Although no specific regulation currently exists in relation to embryonic tissue, the Report notes the recommendations of the Review of the Guidelines on the Research Use of Fetuses and Fetal Material (Polkinghorne Report) [23]. This report argued for caution in the use of such tissue, most specifically in relation to the possibility that abortion decisions might be taken in order that either therapeutic or financial benefits might be obtained. Therefore, Polkinghorne's position – endorsed by the Nuffield Report – was that the decision to terminate a pregnancy must be separate from the decision to permit the use of foetal material in this way. Equally, women intending to donate must be given counselling and adequate information.

It might be thought somewhat surprising that the Nuffield Report did not recommend that legislation should cover this area – particularly as it could be inserted into the abortion legislation every bit as easily as could their other proposed legislative changes. However, it seems that they were satisfied that the guidelines derived from the Polkinghorne Report would be sufficient. Arguably, however, the omission to recommend statutory engagement in this area is serious. Indeed, it could be said that it flies in the face of the general tone of the Report itself, which seems clearly to embrace a statutory framework.

Somatic cell nuclear transfer (SCNT)

In this case, the Nuffield Council notes that similar ethical concerns are raised to those already discussed. However, they also note that there are additional questions connected to this area. Not least, the use of SCNT would require a source of oocytes. Currently, the HFEA has a code of practice in this respect which permits oocytes to be used in research if they have been donated with prior written consent[6]. For the moment, as has been seen, only some kinds of nuclear transfer are directly covered by the Act and the Nuffield Report recommends that the HFEA should take advice on whether or not amendment to the legislation would be needed to cover all potential developments.

Conclusion

For decades, in the UK, there has been a tradition essentially mandating non-interference in medical practice. Beyond legislation designed to create the relevant bodies for self-regulation in medicine, and the intrusion of the Abortion legislation and the Human Fertilisation and Embryology Act, a hands-off approach has been taken. Society thus relies heavily on the judgement and discretion of medicine and science. Arguably, the 1990 Act saw the end of this *laissez faire* approach. The possible uses and misuses of assisted reproductive techniques and technologies, combined with public concern about the services themselves, and in particular concern about the creation, disposition and use of human embryos, tolled the death-knell of total self-regulation, at least in this area.

If for no other reason than to allay public fears, it seems likely that a similar approach needs to be taken in terms of stem cell research. In some cases, it is unarguable that

---

6. http://www.hfea.gov.uk/frame2.htm.

stem cell research differs from currently authorised research only in terms of intended outcome. It is plausible, in fact, to argue that the potential benefits of stem cell research are much greater than those which follow currently permitted human embryo research. The capacity to create tissue for transplantation, for example, would affect an enormous number of people world-wide. Indeed, it may be that the benefits to be derived from stem cell research are considerably greater than the benefits which might be obtained from research into, for example, the causes of infertility. Global, and severe, shortages of organs for donation, for example, could be reduced – perhaps even obviated – if stem cell research leads to the capacity to generate organs. Indeed, stem cell research could lead to effective treatments for a range of human conditions. If this is accepted, then it is difficult to argue for anything other than ensuring its permissibility.

However, for the moment, this is speculation. Animal experiments in stem cell research have not been a major success to date and there is arguably no reason to believe that the translation from animal (once successful) to human is anything other than a long way off. The question, therefore, must be asked: is it either wise or necessary to embrace in ethics or in law the continued development of research in this area, particularly when it involves the use, and the sacrifice, of human embryos? It is not necessary to disapprove of the use of human embryos to take this question seriously. Even those who have no quarrel with human embryo research may feel that it is necessary to draw firm lines in the sand to prevent their over-exposure to research, particularly where there is no clear reason to imagine benefit to be derived from it – at least in the near future.

However, if such research is to continue, the recent critical attention paid to medicine and science – partly as a result of the so-called genetics revolution – makes it imperative that it is regulated, policed and monitored closely. The virtually unanimous, often frightened, world-wide response to the cloning of Dolly, for example, suggests that – even discounting the hysteria and media hype which surrounded this event – there are sound reasons to believe that the public (who should have a voice in these matters) will tolerate no less than this. If this is accepted, then there would seem to be a clear need for revision of the current legislation, to confront next generation research and to locate it within ethically accepted boundaries. Of course, this may mean that some brakes are applied to scientific progress, but – arguably – this is a small price to pay for the clarity and certainty which would accompany it.

Addendum

Since this paper was written, the Government's Chief Medical Officer has reported on this area. Although brief mention of this has been made in the narrative, it might be simpler simply to enumerate their recommendations.

What follows is a direct quotation from the Report, and summarises the conclusions reached:

Recommendations

Recommendation 1

Research using embryos (whether created by *in vitro* fertilisation or cell nuclear replacement) to increase understanding about human disease and disorders and their cell-based treatments should be permitted, subject to the controls in the Human Fertilisation and Embryology Act 1990.

Recommendation 2

In licensing any research using embryos created by cell nuclear replacement, the Human Fertilisation and Embryology Authority should satisfy itself that there are no other means of meeting the objectives of the research.

Recommendation 3

Individuals whose eggs or sperm are used to create the embryos to be used in research should give specific consent indicating whether the resulting embryos could be used in a research project to derive stem cells.

Recommendation 4

Research to increase understanding of, and develop treatments for, mitochondrial diseases using the cell nuclear replacement technique in human eggs, which are subsequently fertilised by human sperm, should be permitted subject to the controls in the Human Fertilisation and Embryology Act 1990.

Recommendation 5

The progress of research involving stem cells which have been derived from embryonic sources should be monitored by an appropriate body to establish whether the research is delivering the anticipated benefits and to identify any concerns which may arise.

Recommendation 6

The mixing of human adult (somatic) cells with the live eggs of any animal species should not be permitted.

Recommendation 7

The transfer of an embryo created by cell nuclear replacement into the uterus of a woman (so called "reproductive cloning") should remain a criminal offence.

Recommendation 8

The need for legislation to permit the use of embryo-derived cells in treatments developed from this new research should be kept under review.

Recommendation 9

The Research Councils should be encouraged to establish a programme for stem cell research and to consider the feasibility of establishing collections of stem cells for research use [24].

References

1. *Human Fertilisation and Embryology Act*, 1990, Schedule 2, S. 3 (1).
2. *Human Fertilisation and Embryology Act*, 1990, Schedule 2, S. 3 (2).
3. *Human Fertilisation and Embryology Act*, 1990, Schedule 2, SS 3 (3) (a) and (4).
4. *Human Fertilisation and Embryology Act*, Code of Practice, December 1995: p. 48 § 10.3.
5. *Human Fertilisation and Embryology Act*, 1990: p. 38 § 7.6.
6. *Human Fertilisation and Embryology Act*, 1990: p. 49 § 10.6.
7. *Human Fertilisation and Embryology Act*, 1990: S. 3 (3) (d).
8. *Stem Cell Therapy: The Ethical Issues*. London, Nuffield Council of Bioethics, April 2000: p. 7 § 15.
9. *Stem Cell Research: Medical Progress with Responsibility*, London, Department of Health. June 2000. Available at http://www.doh.gov.uk/cegc/stemcellreport.pdf.
10. Human Genetics Advisory Commission and the Human Fertilisation and Embryology Authority. *Cloning Issues in Reproduction, Science and Medicine*. London: DTI, 1998.
11. *Stem Cell Therapy: The Ethical Issues*. London, Nuffield Council of Bioethics, April 2000: p. 8 § 21.
12. *Stem Cell Research: Medical Progress with Responsability*, London, Department of Health, June 2000: p. 39 § 4.12. Avaible at http://www.doh.gov.uk/cegc/stemcellreport.pdf.
13. *Stem Cell Therapy: The Ethical Issues*, London, Nuffield Council of Bioethics, April 2000: p. 1.
14. *Stem Cell Therapy: The Ethical Issues*. London, Nuffield Council on Bioethics, April 2000: p. 9 § 22.
15. *Stem Cell Therapy: The Ethical Issues*. London, Nuffield Council on Bioethics, April 2000: p. 4 § 7.
16. *Stem Cell Therapy: The Ethical Issues*. London, Nuffield Council on Bioethics, April 2000: p. 2 § 2.
17. *Stem Cell Research: Medical Progress with Responsibility*. London, Department of Health, June 2000: April 2000, p. 8 § 8. Available at http://www.doh.gov.uk/cegc/stemcellreport.pdf.
18. *Stem Cell Therapy: The Ethical Issues*. London, Nuffield Council on Bioethics, April 2000: p. 9-10 § 25.
19. Mc Lean SAM. *Consultation Document, Consent to Treatment: Review of the Current Provisions of the Human Fertilisation and Embryology Act 1990*, Department of Health 1997.
20. Mc Lean SAM. *Review of the consent provisions of the human fertilisation and embryology Act*, London, Department of Health, July 1998.
21. *Ethical Issues in Human Stem Cell Research:* Volume 1, National Bioethics Advisory Commission, Maryland, USA, 1999.
22. *Stem Cell Therapy: The Ethical Issues*. London, Nuffield Council on Bioethics, April 2000: p. 11 § 28.
23. Cm 762, 1989.
24. *Stem Cell Research: Medical Research: Medical Progress with Responsibility*. London, Department of Health, June 2000: p. 10-11 § 33. Available at http://www.doh.gov.uk/cegc/stemcellreport.pdf.

The moral status of the embryo
and the politics of human stem cell research

Andrew W. Siegel

Bioethics Institute and School of Public Health, Johns Hopkins University, Baltimore, USA

A great deal of fanfare has surrounded the recent announcements of the successful isolation and culturing of human embryonic stem (ES) cells. These pluripotent cells have the capacity to develop into more specialized cells of the human body (*e.g.*, blood, heart, muscle, and brain cells). Research identifying the mechanisms that govern cell differentiation would furnish the foundation for directed differentiation of pluripotent stem cells into specific cell types. The ability to generate specialized cells and tissues would, in turn, significantly advance the development of therapies for treating diseases and injuries.

The tremendous therapeutic promise of ES cell research has inspired a large outpouring of support for the research. However, the research has also met with serious opposition. Opponents of research with stem cells derived from human embryos argue that human embryos have the moral status of persons, and, as such, have a right to life. Since the harvesting of stem cells from embryos results in the destruction of the embryo, researchers who use ES cells are viewed as implicated in the unjust killing of innocent human beings.

The political debate over ES cell research in the United States arises from the conflict between competing views about the moral permissibility of destroying embryos. In this paper, I will discuss the moral and political controversy surrounding ES cell research and seek to mediate the dispute between the opposing parties. I will argue that there is in fact a foundation for a consensus that would allow some research uses of human embryonic stem cells.

The regulation of research with human embryos in the United States

In the United States, research with human embryos and embryonic cell lines that is funded entirely by the private sector is largely unregulated. There are ten states that prohibit or restrict research with *in vitro* embryos[1]. In all other states, scientists may pursue privately funded research uses of embryos without interference from the government. There are, however, strict limitations on federally funded research with human embryos. These limitations are specified in the appropriations bill for the Depart-

---

1. For a summary of state laws on embryo research, see [1].

ment of Health and Human Services (DHHS), which states that no federal funds may be allocated for *"(1) the creation of a human embryo or embryos for research purposes; or (2) research in which a human embryo or embryos are destroyed, discarded, or knowingly subjected to risk or injury or death greater than that allowed for research on fetuses in utero"* [2].

Given that the harvesting of human embryonic stem cells results in the destruction of the embryo, it is clear from the language of the law that federal funds cannot be used to support the derivation of these cells. What has been less clear is whether the law permits federal funding of research uses of the cell lines derived from human embryos. Shortly after the reports of the isolation and culturing of human ES cells, Harold Varmus, then Director of the National Institutes of Health, requested a legal opinion on this issue from the DHHS. Legal counsel for DHHS stated that the law does not apply to research uses of ES cells because (i) these cells are not themselves embryos; and (ii) the statutory language – *"research in which a human embryo or embryos are destroyed"* – refers only to the specific act of destroying an embryo, and does not encompass research that depends upon the prior destruction of an embryo[2]. After receiving this opinion, Dr. Varmus set up a committee to establish guidelines for federally funded human stem cell research. The final guidelines, published on August 23, 2000, prohibit federal funding of the derivation of human embryonic stem cells but permit federal funding of research uses of the cells under the following conditions [3]:

– the embryos from which the stem cells were derived were produced by *in vitro* fertilization for fertility treatment, were in excess of the clinical needs of those seeking treatment, were frozen prior to donation, and had not reached the stage of mesodermal formation ;
– the individuals undergoing fertility treatment gave informed consent for the use of their embryos in stem cell research, and they were not approached about consenting to donate their embryos for stem cell research prior to the time of deciding the disposition of the excess embryos ;
– no inducements were offered for the donation of embryos for research ;
– the donation of embryos was not made with any limits or specification concerning who may be a recipient of transplantation of cells derived from the embryos ;
– researchers must obtain the cells through a donation or a payment that *"does not exceed the reasonable costs associated with the transportation, processing, preservation, quality control and storage of the cells"* ;
– researchers must not utilize the cells to *"create or contribute to a human embryo"*.

While NIH plans to begin reviewing grant applications for research with human ES cells soon, some legislators have asserted that any federal support of this research would be in violation of the law. A large number of Congressmen involved in the passage of the law restricting funding of embryo research maintain that DHHS misinterpreted the law in reading it as covering only the act of destroying a human embryo. According to these legislators, the law was also meant to *"bar the use of tax dollars to fund research which follows or depends upon the destruction of or injury to a human embryo"*[3]. Thus, on this interpretation, it is illegal to federally fund the use or derivation

---
2. Memorandum from Harriet Rabb, General Counsel at HHS, to Harold Varmus (January 15, 1999).
3. Letter from seventy members of Congress to Donna Shalala, Secretary of Health and Human Services (February 11, 1999).

of ES cells. Because NIH has rejected this interpretation, some Congressmen are proposing legislation that would explicitly ban all federal support of human ES cell research.

At the same time, there are legislators and others calling for federal funding of both the derivation and use of ES cells. President Clinton's National Bioethics Advisory Commission (NBAC) recommended this and cited several grounds for federally funding the derivation of ES cells:

"First, researchers using human ES cell lines will derive substantial benefits from a detailed understanding of the process of ES cell derivation, because the properties of ES cells and the methods for sustaining the cell lines may differ depending upon the conditions and methods used to derive them... Second, significant basic research must be conducted regarding the process of ES cell derivation before cell-based therapies can be fully realized... Third, ES cells are not indefinitely stable in culture. As these cells are grown, irreversible changes occur in their genetic makeup. Thus... it is important to be able to repeatedly derive ES cells in order to ensure that the properties of the cells that are being studied have not changed" [4].

President Clinton has not supported NBAC's recommendation to fund the derivation of ES cells. But he has embraced the NIH guidelines, and remarked that the guidelines *"meet rigorous ethical standards"* [5].

Derivation, use, and ethical consistency

We might, however, question whether a policy that draws a sharp line between the derivation and use of embryonic stem cells satisfies the requirements of ethical rigor. Consider, for the moment, the perspective of those who assert that the human embryo has the moral status of a person. On this view, the derivation of ES cells is clearly morally problematic, as it involves the destruction of the embryo. But researchers who use stem cells that others have derived will also generally be seen as in connivance in the destruction of embryos. From this perspective, researchers who enlist the services of others to perform the derivation of stem cells are rather like those who collaborate with hit men to accomplish their ends. While their hands may not be as dirty as those of the individuals who destroy the embryos, these researchers are nonetheless regarded as very much implicated in the demise of the embryos.

There may be circumstances in which opponents of ES cell research could not properly deem researchers who use ES cells morally responsible for the destruction of embryos. Suppose, for example, that a researcher, X, accepts an unsolicited donation of a cell line from another investigator, Y, who created the cell line for her own research. Is X at all culpable for Y's derivation of ES cells? One might hold that we cannot assign moral responsibility for the destruction of embryos to investigators like X because, as John Robertson puts it, their *"research plans or actions had no effect on whether the original immoral derivation occurred"* [6]. On the other hand, while these investigators may not be responsible for the destruction of the particular embryos from which the cell lines were derived, they might still be viewed as implicated in the destruction of embryos more generally by virtue of their being participants in a research enterprise that creates a demand for the derivation of ES cells and contributes to the legitimation of the practice. Even if it sometimes is not possible to hold investigators who use ES cells responsible for the destruction of embryos, opponents of the research would likely consider investigators in such instances to be tainted by a symbolic association with the practice.

In any case, it is evident that much research with ES cells will be morally tied to the derivation of the cells. The moral link between the use and derivation of ES cells casts doubt upon the justifiability of the current US policy on ES cell research. The interpretation of the law on embryo research that informs the NIH guidelines is problematic because it fails to consider the moral purpose animating the ban on federal funding of embryo research. In considering whether research with ES cells constitutes *"research in which human embryos are destroyed"*, it is not sufficient to appeal, as some defenders of the DHHS opinion do, to the fact that *"there is no indication that either proponents or opponents contemplated the situation under consideration here, in which research that destroyed the embryo was separately conducted from research using the cells derived from the embryo"* [7]. As H.L.A. Hart has noted, *"in no legal system is the scope of legal rules restricted to the range of concrete instances which were present or are believed to have been present in the minds of legislators"* [8]. Instead, one has to look at the more general legislative purpose(s) underlying a law. In the present case, it is clear from the whole debate surrounding human embryo research that the enactment of the ban on human embryo research was motivated by a moral concern about respect for human life. The law can reasonably be viewed as embodying the principle that the federal government should not be implicated in the intentional destruction of innocent human life. Since, as discussed above, researchers who use ES cells will typically be implicated in the destruction of human embryos, it is reasonable to interpret the embryo research law as prohibiting federal funding of research with ES cells.

Given the moral links between the use and derivation of ES cells, those who wish to promote a policy permitting federal funding of research uses of ES cells must defend the derivation of the cells. This requires a defense of the destruction of human embryos for ES cell research. There are two general strategies one might pursue in seeking to furnish this account. One approach is to provide a moral argument that supports the destruction of embryos. The other approach is to offer a political argument supporting the destruction of embryos that is neutral on the issue of the morality of the act. I shall argue below that the latter approach offers the most promising strategy for defending federal support of ES cell research.

The moral case for ES cell research

The most straightforward moral case for permitting the destruction of human embryos for ES cell research is an utilitarian one. An utilitarian could argue that the sacrifice of human embryos is justified by the tremendous therapeutic benefits ES cell research is likely to generate. But while no one would question the value of promoting good social consequences, there are constraints on the kinds of actions we can take to advance the social good. It is, for example, impermissible to intentionally kill innocent persons or experiment on persons without their informed consent, even if it would sometimes maximize net utility to do such things. Opponents of ES cell research hold that the moral rule against intentionally killing innocent persons to advance the common good extends to our treatment of human embryos. According to opponents of the research, human embryos have the same moral status as children and adult humans, with a right to life that cannot be sacrificed for the benefit of society. Thus, the moral case for ES cell research requires more than an appeal to the potential benefits of the research. One must also rebut the claim that human embryos have the moral status of persons.

It is, however, notoriously difficult to furnish satisfactory criteria for moral personhood. Those who deny the personhood of embryos typically identify cognitive or psychological capacities that are thought essential to personhood but which embryos lack. The most commonly cited capacities include consciousness, self-consciousness, and reasoning [9-11]. The problem with such accounts is that they appear to be either under- or over-inclusive, depending on which capacities are invoked. If self-consciousness or reasoning is essential to personhood, then most early infants will not count as persons. If sentience is the touchstone of the right to life, then non human animals will also possess this right. Since most of those who reject the personhood of the embryo believe that newborn infants do possess a right to life and animals do not, we cannot generally appeal to these capacities to morally distinguish embryos from other human beings.

Those who reject that embryos have the moral status of persons might simply claim that the embryo is too nascent a form of human life to merit the respect accorded to more developed humans. But in the absence of an account that decisively identifies the first stage of development at which moral personhood begins, it is not possible to establish that human embryos do not possess a right to life.

The history of the debate on personhood certainly suggests that a resolution of the matter is not soon forthcoming. Those who support ES cell research would do well to argue their case without attempting to settle the debate over the moral status of embryos. Ideally, the justification for federal funding of the research should be one that individuals with opposing views on the status of the embryo can accept. As A. Gutmann and D. Thompson argue, the construction of public policy on morally controversial issues should involve a *"search for significant points of convergence between one's own understanding and those of citizens whose positions, taken in their more comprehensive forms, one must reject"* [12].

A political argument for federal funding of ES cell research

A political justification for funding of ES cell research must be neutral on the question of the moral status of the embryo, and seek its foundation instead in an overlapping consensus between competing moral views about the embryo. Of course, as long as the debate is understood strictly in terms of a dispute between those who believe the embryo has the moral status of a person and those who think the embryo has little or no moral standing, it will not be possible to discover an overlapping consensus. But I believe this is a misleading portrayal of the conflict. Once we recognize this, it will be evident that there is sufficient consensus on the status of embryos to justify some federal funding of ES cell research.

There are grounds for supposing that a large faction of conservatives who oppose the destruction of embryos do not in fact believe that the human embryo is a person with a right to life. Consider the exceptions to the prohibition on federal funding of abortions that most of these conservatives support. Federal funding of abortion is prohibited except in cases of rape and incest, and where abortion is necessary to save the life of the mother [13]. These exceptions reflect a common sentiment amongst conservatives about the conditions under which abortion is morally permissible. Yet, these exceptions seem incompatible with the view that the foetus is a person with a right to life.

With respect to the rape and incest exceptions, it would, as Ronald Dworkin comments, be *"contradictory to insist that a foetus has a right to live that is strong enough to justify prohibiting abortion even when childbirth would ruin a mother's or a family's life, but that ceases to exist when the pregnancy is the result of a sexual crime of which the foetus is, of course, wholly innocent"* [14]. In instances where abortion is necessary to save the mother's life, it does not seem that one who regards the foetus as a person would have good reason to privilege the mother's life over the foetus's life. Indeed, inasmuch as the mother typically bears some responsibility for putting the foetus in the position in which it needs her aid, one who regards the foetus as a person might well hold that the foetus's life should be privileged. Suppose, for example, that X and Y are hanging off the side of a cliff as a result of a negligent act of X's, and it is only possible to save one of their lives. One might reasonably hold that Y has a stronger claim to assistance than X. Certainly, Y has at least an equal claim to assistance. Likewise, if one supposes that the foetus is a person, its right to aid is equal to or greater than the mother's right to aid in cases where one of their lives must be sacrificed to save the other.

The significance of these exceptions in the context of ES cell research is that they suggest we can identify a foundation for consensus between liberals and conservatives on the permissibility of destroying embryos. Conservatives who allow these exceptions implicitly hold with liberals that very early forms of human life can sometimes be sacrificed to advance the interests of other humans. Although liberals and conservatives will disagree about the range of ends for which human embryos can be destroyed, they should be able to reach some consensus. Conservatives who hold that it is permissible to kill a foetus in order to save a pregnant woman or spare a rape victim additional trauma ought to concur with liberals that it is permissible to destroy embryos where there is good reason to believe that it is necessary to save lives or prevent extreme suffering.

Given the great promise of ES cell research for the fight against life-threatening and severely debilitating diseases, the consensus that liberals and conservatives should be able to arrive at on the destruction of embryos appears sufficient to warrant federal funding of the derivation and use of ES cells. Thus, there are grounds for changing the current federal law on funding of embryo research. It is important to note, however, that the consensus identified above is consistent with the current ban on federally funding the creation of embryos for research purposes. For one who accepts that it is sometimes permissible to sacrifice an embryo originally produced for procreative purposes (or a foetus created by mistake or force) to advance the interests of other humans need not find it acceptable to create an embryo with the intention of destroying it.

There are several objections one might pose to the argument presented here, none of which I think are compelling. Some might claim that the abortion exceptions do not provide an adequate foundation for consensus on embryo research. One could argue that the abortion and embryo research cases are morally distinct inasmuch the existence of a foetus directly conflicts with the pregnant woman's interests, while a particular *ex utero* embryo does not threaten anyone's interests. But this distinction does not bear much moral weight, as it is the implicit attribution of greater value to the interests of adult humans over any interests the foetus may have that informs the judgment that it is permissible to kill it in the cases at issue. One might also argue that the benefits of ES cell research are too uncertain to justify a comparison with abortion. But the lower probability of benefits from ES cell research is balanced by a high ratio of potential lives saved for lives lost. Finally, there are those who maintain that the ES cell research is unnecessary because adult stem cells can be used to achieve the same ends. But while recent findings suggest adult stem cells are more versatile than previously thought, ES cells presently appear to be a superior source of cells and tissues because of, *inter alia*, their capacity to proliferate indefinitely in the laboratory without changing properties. This is, however, a matter that must continually be revisited by policymakers as the research progresses. There is at least reason to hope that scientific and technological advances will ultimately eliminate the ethical and political strife surrounding human stem cell research.

References

1. Lori A. State regulation of embryo stem cell research. In: *Ethical issues in human stem cell research*. Volume II of the National Bioethics Commission Report. January 2000.
2. Public Law 105-277, section 511(a) (1) & (2).
3. National Institutes of Health Guidelines for research using human pluripotent stem cells. August 25, 2000.
4. National Bioethics Advisory Commission. *Ethical issues in human stem cell research*. Volume I, September 1999: p. 71.
5. Hopper DI. *Clinton touts embryo research rules*. Associated Press, August 23, 2000.
6. Robertson J. Ethics and policy in embryonic stem cell research. *Kennedy Inst Ethics J* 1999; 9 (2): 109-36.
7. Flannery EJ, Javitt GH. Analysis of federal laws pertaining to funding of human pluripotent stem cell research. In: *Ethical issues in human stem cell research*. Volume II of the National Bioethics Commission Report. January 2000.
8. Hart HLA. Positivism and the separation of law and morals. 71 *Harvard Law Review* 593, 1958.
9. Feinberg J. Abortion. In: Regan T, ed. *Matters of life and death*, 1986: 256-93.
10. Tooley M. *Abortion and infanticide*, 1983.
11. Warren MA. On the moral and legal status of abortion. *The Monist* 1973; 57: 43-61.
12. Gutmann A, Thompson D. *Democracy and Disagreement*, 1996.
13. Title V, Labor, HHS, and Education Appropriations, 112 Stat. 3681-385, Sec. 509(a) (1) & (2).
14. Dworkin R. *Life's Dominion*, 1994: 32.

Are all cells derived from an embryo themselves embryos?

Norman Ford
Caroline Chisholm Centre for Health Ethics, Melbourne, Australia

Once human embryos were only formed by fertilisation when egg and sperm fuse at syngamy to generate a new life in the first cell, the zygote. Now there are other ways. I believe that any human embryo ought to be treated as a person because there are reasonable grounds to believe the human individual is present from conception. I also hold it would be unethical to use or to benefit from the use of cells obtained by collusion with the destruction of embryos. In this chapter, I do not argue this case, but instead I take it for granted.

Since the beginning of *in vitro* fertilisation (IVF) human embryos have been formed outside the body. With more opportunities for experimentation on embryos questions arise about what is to count as an embryo. Embryos can be disaggregated and cells can be removed from an embryo for preimplantation diagnosis or manipulated for research. It is necessary, then, to know when an embryo is created or destroyed by these techniques. For ethical and legal reasons, a definition is needed for the due protection of artificially formed human embryos. Before attempting this, a review of some facts about natural and artificial ways of forming embryos would be helpful.

Following six cell divisions some four days after fertilisation the 64 or so compacted cells of the morula form the early blastocyst. Its outer cells are destined to become extraembryonic membranes and placental tissue, while many, but not all, of the cell progeny of the inner cell mass (ICM) are destined to form the fetus. Contact and induction signals between the ICM and trophoblast cells are essential for continued organised species specific human development, to generate a body plan and to complete implantation[1].

Trophoblast cells can be removed from the blastocyst leaving the ICM isolated. This raises questions about the status of the cells of an embryo following its disaggregation. Is the ICM in this situation still an embryo? Are trophoblast cells an embryo? After the ICM cells are treated to grow and multiply in culture, they are usually called embryonic stem (ES) cells or pluripotent stem cells. Are ES cells embryos? Is a cry-

---

1. For more details see [1, p. 151-6].

opreserved embryo still an embryo? Does somatic nuclear transfer to an enucleated egg result in the generation of an embryo after the cell is reprogrammed and activated? Does parthenogenetic activation of an egg create an embryo?

Potential for development

An egg is not an embryo, but egg and sperm have the potential to generate or become an embryo at fertilisation. An embryo has actual and active potential to continue development. Freezing an embryo suspends metabolic activity and development [1, p. 155]. Frozen embryos are not dead but dormant, living in suspended animation. They retain their actual potential for human development which resumes after thawing.

It is sometimes said that all totipotent cells are embryos. This needs clarification. In the strong meaning of the term, a totipotent embryo has the actual potential to produce the blastocyst, placental tissues and entire offspring. The use of totipotency with this meaning provides grounds for the moral status of an embryo. In a weak sense, totipotency is also used to refer to the actual capacity of the progeny of one or more embryonic cells to form all types of cells, but they cannot produce an entire embryo or fetus. These cells are also called pluripotent stem cells.

Manipulated embryos

The timing of blastulation and the minimum number of cells required for it is species specific [2]. If there are too few cells, blastulation cannot occur because there would not be enough cells to form the inner cell mass (ICM) and the outer cells. Sometimes the ICM splits *in vivo* and forms identical twin or triplet embryos which survive because they all use the existing trophoblast tissue and eventual placenta. But if half of an artificially isolated ICM is promptly surrounded by trophoblast cells, it would probably survive after transfer to the uterus in the same way as an identical twin. By day six the ICM and trophoblast cells of a blastocyst are clearly distinct, with a total of about 168 cells if they are grown in sequential culture media [3]. The excising of the trophoblast cells from the ICM of a blastocyst and placing the ICM in culture eventually destroy the blastocyst/embryo. Although these ICM cells may still divide, their progeny are no longer part of organised species specific human development because they lack the necessary contact with sufficient trophoblast cells. At this point they are deemed to be ES cells because they simply multiply in culture and cannot receive induction signals generated by the "inside-outside" contact mechanism.

However, if a two-cell human embryo is split, each cell can continue species specific human development and identical twin offspring can be formed after each cell is placed in an empty zona pellucida (ZP) and transferred to the uterus. The same would apply to each half or quarter of a four, – eight – or sixteen-cell embryo. Blastulation would occur about the same time in all cases – about four days after fertilisation. It seems that blastulation is governed by a "clock mechanism", in-built into the DNA of each cell of the embryo from fertilisation [1, p. 155, 158, 174-5, 206].

Research with sheep embryos shows that when a cell is isolated from a four-cell embryo, placed in an empty ZP and transferred to the uterus, its cell progeny can develop normally. This means a cell excised from a four-cell embryo could become a new embryo. The same might also apply to a single cell from an eight-cell embryo [1, p. 139-41]. However, if a single cell were to be excised from a sixteen-cell embryo and placed in a ZP, its cell progeny would attempt to blastulate at the preset time. But this cell would come from the fourth division and attempted blastulation would occur after two-three divisions. As a result blastulation would fail as there would not be enough cells to form the ICM and outer cells of the blastocyst.

Human ICM cells have now been isolated and grown in culture on a feeder layer where they flatten out as ES cells and thereby lose the organisation of an embryo. They can continue to divide without differentiating for months [4]. After Dolly's birth, scientists realised that even in mammals, after a somatic cell nucleus is fused with an enucleated egg, it can be re-programmed to the undifferentiated state. Following activation, development is started and a cloned embryo may be formed [5]. So far, nobody has produced an embryo from ES cells in primates. At present ES cells can only be obtained from embryos, but it may be possible in the future to obtain them artificially from another source, *e.g.* the partial reversal of differentiation of adult somatic cells to the pluripotent, but not the totipotent stage [6].

A mouse egg can be stimulated to begin development by an electric shock without being fertilised by sperm – this is known as parthenogenesis. Parthenogenetic development can only go on to mid-gestation (10 days) or even up to 13 days because sperm contribution is needed for proper embryonic and placental development [1, p. 107, 149-51] [7, 8]. Until death, however, the fetus would be a parthenogenetic mouse developed from an egg alone.

Finally, in an experiment, András Nagy and his colleagues sandwiched mouse ES cells between the trophoblast cells of non-viable tetraploid embryos to test their developmental potential. Chimaeric aggregation embryos were formed. After their transfer to recipient females, live mice were born which were genetically derived from the ES cells [9][2].

Definition of an embryo

Reflection on the process of human development as well as on the case of a frozen embryo suggests the following definition of a human embryo: a single-cell, or multicellular, organism which has the inherent actual potential to continue species specific, *i.e.* typical, human development, given a suitable environment. This implies typical development must begin. It does not mean that an embryo affected by Down's syndrome or even a lethal congenital abnormality such as trisomy 18 is not a human embryo. Rather, the product of an unsuccessful attempt at fertilisation that is inherently incapable of forming a developing zygote is not an embryo. Embryonic tumours and teratomas

---

2. Nagy *et al.* stated: *"In such chimeras, the tetraploid component is selected against in all lineages where ES cells are able to differentiate normally following the ES cells to take over the embryo proper and relegating the tetraploid component to the extraembryonic membranes [9, p. 8424]."*

are not embryos because they are not organisms with the requisite actual potential to continue species specific human development.

Some cells derived from an embryo are not embryos

In light of what happens in sheep, it may be assumed that a single cell isolated from a 2-8 cell human embryo would become a new embryo and could develop to term if placed in an empty ZP and then in a uterus [1, p. 140-1]. But an isolated cell from a 16-32-cell morula would lack the actual potential for typical human development and would not be an embryo.

When the trophoblast cells are removed from a human blastocyst, leaving an isolated ICM, the blastocyst does not survive. For argument's sake, if a whole isolated ICM were to be promptly surrounded with sufficient trophoblast cells from another embryo it could be said that the original embryo-blastocyst from which the ICM was taken would continue to survive after being implanted in the uterus. In other words, this could be compared to a rescue operation of the same embryo. By analogy with the formation of human twins and triplets by the splitting of the ICM *in vivo*, it could be assumed a half or a third of an isolated ICM could likewise be rescued by enveloping them with sufficient trophoblast cells before implanting them in the uterus. I am not suggesting anybody should do this, but it does show that an embryo does not definitively cease to exist as soon as the trophoblast cells are excised from the blastocyst. This is because an isolated ICM would still retain its actual potential to continue typical human development and would continue to do so once it is rescued, in much the same way as a frozen embryo continues development after thawing out. However, once an ICM is placed in culture and its cells begin to spread out and multiply, they promptly lose their organisation and actual potential for typical development and become ES cells.

Instances of human parthenogenetic development have been reported in IVF [10]. Granted a parthenogenetic mouse fetus is derived from a mouse egg, we would have to admit that IVF parthenogenetic embryos develop from human eggs following their activation by electric shock. Assuming typical development occurs, they would be human embryos until they perish. This, however, does not imply a human egg is an embryo. An egg has the potential to become an embryo, but not prior to activation followed by typical human development.

As regards nuclear transfer, it remains unknown whether somatic nuclear transfer to an enucleated egg would succeed to form an embryo in the human. If it did, a cloned human embryo would be formed.

In the light of Nagy's experiment, it is asked whether human ES cells are embryos or their equivalents? James Thomson and Vivienne Marshall commented as follows:

"It is not known whether human ES cells could form a complete, viable embryo by any method, but this possibility has raised the greatest concern about the derivation of human ES cells [11][3]*."*

---

3. On the same page they continued: *"Although the ES cells have the potential to differentiate to any cell in the body, the cells are not the equivalent of an intact embryo. If a clump of ES cells were transferred to*

Nicholas Tonti-Filipinni and Peter McCullagh note that Nagy's experiment shows that mouse ES cells are totipotent in the strong sense: *"ES cells taken from a blastocyst can form a whole mouse* [12]*."* They suggest that the trophoblast cells favour development and growth rather than adding a capacity for embryological development that was not intrinsic to the nature of the ES cells [12]. While recognising it is not in fact known whether a human being could be derived from ES cells, they clearly state:

On the evidence available now, there would appear to be a reasonably good chance that human ES cells could, if suitably manipulated, develop into embryos [12].

Similar views were expressed during a hearing of an Australian Federal Government Inquiry into Human Cloning[4].

An alternative view is that neither a single ES cell nor a clump of ES cells satisfy the conditions required to be an embryo. They are not the same embryo/blastocyst from which they are derived nor are they a new embryo. Furthermore the original ICM cells can multiply to form hundreds of ES cells in culture. ES cells are not an organism with actual potential for typical human development as in the case of a freshly isolated ICM discussed above. Evidence is lacking for a clump of ES cells to be an organism. In a recent study of human ES cells, Benjamin Reubinoff reported:

"In [these] high-density cultures, there was no consistent pattern of structural organisation suggestive of the formation of embryoid bodies similar to those formed in mouse ES cell aggregates or arising sporadically in marmoset ES cell cultures... There was no evidence of growth or formation of distinct tissue layers in the aggregates. When the surviving clumps were replated on to tissue culture plastic in standard medium culture cell death was evident, and no extensive outgrowth occurred. Thus, manipulations used in our laboratory and elsewhere to facilitate embryoid body formation and multilineage differentiation of mouse ES cells induced death of human ES cells [13]*."*

The source embryo and the ICM cease to exist by the time ES cells flatten out in culture without organisation and begin to multiply. The original embryo cannot be rescued if it no longer exists. I do not believe Nagy's experiment provides reasonable grounds to believe mouse ES cells become a mouse embryo before their aggregation with trophoblast cells from another mouse embryo. Without surrounding trophoblast cells a clump of ES cells could not become an embryo which can begin and continue typical human development. However, the possibility could not be excluded that a clump of human ES cells could become an embryo once it is wrapped in trophoblast

---

a uterus, the ES cells would not form a viable fetus. Chimeras formed from mouse cells and tetraploid embryos allow the formation of a complete viable fetus by the ES cell component in some cases [9], *but it is not known whether this would be biologically possible with human ES cells."*

4. Archbishop Hickey, on behalf of the Australian Catholic Bishops Conference, made the following statement in Canberra on March 2000 at a public hearing of the House of Representatives Standing Committee on Legal and Constitutional Affairs. *Inquiry into the Scientific, Ethical and Regulatory Considerations Relevant to the Cloning of Human Beings*: "Embryonic stem cells should be treated and accorded the respect, and the proper protection, due to a human embryo. There is significant scientific reason to believe that, given certain conditions, totipotent human ES cells may develop into embryos." See the Internet Homepage site: http:www.aph.gov.au/house/committee/laca or http:www.aph.gov.au/hansard.

cells and implanted in a suitable uterine environment. Even in this case, human ES cells would not become an embryo prior to their aggregation with trophoblast cells.

Serious difficulties would arise if we were to accept that a clump of human ES cells is an embryo simply because, given certain conditions, it may become an embryo. A human egg, after artificial activation, may become an embryo. But this does not provide any reasonable grounds to hold that an egg is an embryo. Again, granted the success of somatic nuclear transfer in some mammals, we could assume a human somatic nucleus might also become a cloned human embryo in the same way. But this does not mean that a somatic cell nucleus could be regarded as a human embryo if, after appropriate manipulation, it may become an embryo. An egg has the potential to become an embryo but not before this potential is actualised by fertilisation by sperm or artificial parthenogenetic activation. A somatic cell nucleus has the potential to become an embryo, but not before this potential is actualised by the use of cloning technology.

Serious misunderstandings can arise from the way the term "develop" is sometimes employed in descriptive scientific discourse. A crucial philosophical distinction is to be made between cells that change to become a human embryo, and an embryo that develops into a fetus and a child. At fertilisation egg and sperm become an embryo. The same applies to an egg following parthenogenetic activation. When a clump of ES cells are enveloped in trophoblast cells, they can become a new developing embryo. By means of the cloning technique used for Dolly, the nucleus of a body cell and an enucleated egg can become an embryo. When an embryo and fetus develop, the same entity develops and grows.

Conclusion

An entity is an embryo because of what it is with its actual potential, not because of what it may become. Once an embryo is disaggregated and loses its actual potential for typical development it ceases to exist even if some ES cells live on in culture and multiply. The Infertility Treatment Authority of Victoria has recently stated: *"For the purposes of the Infertility Treatment Act 1995, ES cells are neither gametes nor embryos* [14].*"* The challenge for scientists is to find an ethical way to obtain ES or pluripotent stem cells for medical purposes *without using human* eggs for cloning human embryos or harming human embryos [15]. This may take quite some time. Another promising possibility without ethical problems is to find and induce human adult stem cells to become different kinds of cells useful for therapeutic purposes [16, 17].

Addendum

Reverend Norman Ford SDB wishes to conclude with the timely warning against cloning human embryos given by Pope John Paul II to the 18th International Congress of the Transplant Society in Rome on 29 August 2000 – without reference to any intrinsic value of ES cells themselves:

"Methods that fail to respect the dignity and value of the person must always be avoiled. I am thinking in particular of attempts at human cloning with a view to ob-

taining organs for transplants: these techniques, insofar as they involve the manipulation and destruction of human embryos, are not morally acceptable, even when their proposed goal is good in itself. Science itself points to other forms of therapeutic intervention which would not involve cloning or the use of embryonic cells, but would rather make use of stem cells taken from adults. This is the direction that research must follow if it wishes to respect the dignity of each and every human being, even at the embryonic stage.

In addressing these varied issues, the contribution of philosophers and theologians is important. Their careful and competent reflection on the ethical problems associated with transplant therapy can help to clarify the criteria for assessing what kinds of transplants are morally acceptable and under what conditions, especially with regard to the protection of each individual's personal identity" [18].

References

1. Ford NM. When did I begin? *Conception of the human individual in history, philosophy and science.* Cambridge: University Press, 1991.
2. McLaren A. The embryo. In: Austin CR, Short RV, eds. *Embryonic and fetal development.* Book 2: *Reproduction in mammals.* Cambridge: University Press, 1982.
3. Bongso A. *Handbook on blastocyst culture.* Singapore: National University of Singapore, 1999: 77.
4. Thomsom JA, *et al.* Embryonic stem cell lines derived from human blastocysts. *Science* 1998; 282: 1145-7.
5. Wilmut I, *et al.* Viable offspring derived from fetal and adult mammalian cells. *Nature* 1997; 385: 810-3.
6. Australian Academy of Science. *On human cloning: a position statement.* Canberra, 1999: 15.
7. Kono T, *et al.* Epigenetic modification during oocyte growth correlates with extended parthenogenetic development in the mouse. *Nature Genet* 1996; 13 (1): 91-4.
8. Strum KS, *et al.* Abnormal development of embryonic and extraembryonic cell lineages in parthenogenetic mouse embryos. *Dev Dynamics* 1994; 201 (1): 11-28.
9. Nagy A, *et al.* Derivation of completely cell culture-derived mice from early-passage embryonic stem cells. *Proc Natl Acad Sci USA* 1993; 90: 8428-8.
10. Angell RR, *et al.* Chromosome abnormalities in human embryos after *in vitro* fertilization. *Nature* 1983; 303: 336-8.
11. Thomson JA, Marshall VS. Primate embryonic stem cells. *Curr Top Dev Biol* 1998; 38: 158.
12. Tonti-Filipinni N, McCullagh P. Embryonic stem cells and totipotency. *Ethics & Medics* 2000; 25: 2-3.
13. Reubinoff BE, *et al.* Embryonic stem cell lines from human blastocysts somatic differentiation *in vitro. Nature Biotech* 2000; 18: 401.
14. ITA news. The use of embryonic stem cells. May 2000.
15. Coghlan A. Cloning without embryos. *New Scientist.* January 2000.
16. Alison MR, *et al.* Hepatocytes from non-hepatic adult stem cells. *Nature* 2000; 406: 257.
17. Bjornson CRR, *et al.* A hematopoietic fate adapted by adult neural stem cells *in vivo. Science* 1999; 534: 7.
18. John Paul II. *L'Osservatore Romano.* Weekly Edition in English, 30 August 2000.

Discussion

Marissa Vicari
Mapi Research Institute, Lyon, France

While technological breakthroughs in the field of stem cell research promise significant therapeutic application, they also raise a plethora of ethical and regulatory questions. Much discussion on the ethical aspects of stem cell research has focused on the derivation of human embryonic stem (ES) cells from the human embryo, and the subsequent destruction of the embryo as a result. The central ethical dilemma here concerns the ethical standing and legal statute of the embryo; a topic which in the past has been debated at length in the context of abortion, *in vitro* fertilisation (IVF) technology and prenatal diagnosis.

As in the past, scientific discovery concerning the embryo gives us cause to revisit the philosophical and religious debates on when life begins, what it means to be a person and what our rights and duties as such are. In the context of stem cell research, there are new elements to consider, such as the promise of tremendous benefit to society that may be realised with the development of therapies derived from stem cells, as well as the multiple ways of creating embryos and deriving stem cells. National legislation regarding the use of the embryo in research varies from country to country; thus raising the question "who will develop these technologies and who will benefit from them?"

One aim of incorporating a session on regulation and ethics into this conference, therefore, was to facilitate discussion between bioethicists, regulators and researchers towards the harmonisation of regulations relating to ES cell research and therapeutics. Similar fora have taken place in recent years, in parallel with the development of stem cell research and cloning, to foster the exchange of ideas within a multidiciplinary group. While the panel for this session on ethical issues is by no means representative of the international debate, it presents a multidisciplinary and international approach. Panellists were asked to provide national perspectives, and five countries were represented: France, the United States (USA), the United Kingdom (UK), Germany and Australia. The following discussion will not attempt to summarise the excellent papers presented, rather it is based on points raised by the panellists and participants during the conference.

What is an embryo?

Beginning with definitions, one of the major tasks facing both scientists and regulators is to determine what exactly counts as an embryo and how it relates to the stem cell, considering that stem cells may be derived from embryos of different origin (abortion, *in vitro* fertilisation, cell nuclear transfer) as well as from adult organisms. The developmental potential of stem cells is also a factor that informs our understanding of their relation to the embryo.

As Rev. Norman Ford points out, the scientific terminology of "totipotent" and "pluripotent" stem cells needs clarification. For example, if *"an entity is an embryo because of what it is with its actual potential"* [1], and a "totipotent" stem cell is a cell with the actual potential to produce an entire embryo, then this "totipotent" stem cell could be considered by some as being an embryo in itself. On the other hand, if the term "totipotent" may be used to refer to the capacity of a cell to produce many types of cells *but not* an entire embryo, then this has different implications for research with such "totipotent" stem cells. One perspective, for example, is that the human embryo ought to be treated as a person because there are *"reasonable grounds to believe the human individual is present from conception"* [1]. However, how can we understand conception, and thus the creation of a new embryo, within the context of cell nuclear transfer? This underlies the ethical and legal issue raised by Rev. Ford's chapter, that a definition of *"what counts as an embryo"* is needed *"for the due protection of artificially formed human embryos"* [1].

Is the scientific definition, however, necessarily the appropriate one? In the scientific sessions of this conference, we saw that an incumbent task for researchers is characterising the stem cell itself, that is, providing a descriptive answer to the question "what is a stem cell?" Furthermore, we saw evidence that the plasticity of stem cells might be greater than thought before and that the line between totipotent and pluripotent stem cells may not be definitive. It may be said that the definition of these scientific terms, like our understanding of what they describe, is evolving and will continue to evolve with future research.

In addition, applying definitions from one field to another may not have the desired effect of rendering clarity, due to the fact that definitions in different fields are designed to serve different purposes. Indeed, the scientific definition of the stem cell is based on objective description derived from certain measurements, while the definition offered by Rev. Ford above is concerned with the creation of the individual, which remains a more subjective concept, despite scientific rigor. The legal definition should have the primary aim of clarity, while content follows as a secondary aim. An ever-evolving definition, thus, would be inappropriate for the legal sphere, just as a very clear and stable definition at this time may not be appropriate, or even possible, in the scientific sphere. Neither, of course, would it be appropriate for the regulator to base a legal definition on the beliefs of one group of people, rather the role of the legislator is to represent society as a whole in finding a way to regulate that represents a consensus or compromise.

ES cells and organ donation

Can the donation of supernumerary *in vitro* fertilisation (IVF) embryos be considered in a similar way, on the ethical and regulatory levels, as organ donation? The answer to this question depends on the country considered. In France, for example, this would not be possible because the legal concept of donation supposes consent of the donor, and French regulations specify that one can neither donate for a third party nor can one donate anything other than an object. This is reflected in the terminology used in the French legislation with regard to the "donation" of IVF embryos from one couple to another, where we speak of the reception or welcoming ("accueil") of the embryo by a receiving couple. This case brings us back to the issue of definition since the embryo is legally an individual and not an object, the term donation is actually inappropriate when speaking about couples wanting to "donate" their embryos in France. "Donation" of an embryo, in France, implies objectification of the embryo, which is strictly prohibited under the concept of human dignity. Furthermore, due to the line of reasoning between the principle of consent and organ donation, where we speak of organs (considered as objects) being donated with consent of the donor, "donation" of the embryo, then, presumes that the embryo itself is consenting to be donated, which of course is not possible.

The situation in the UK regarding the understanding of embryo donation is entirely different. As addressed in Sheila McLean's presentation [2], the Nuffield Council reported that the donation, for research purposes, of IVF embryos that will not be implanted is not an act which is disrespectful to the embryos themselves. Rather, the Nuffield Council considers such a donation as being similar to tissue donation. The UK's Chief Medical Officer's report of June, 2000, also upheld that IVF embryos may be donated for research purposes.

In the USA, the donation of embryos is largely unregulated, however, there is a strong feeling that the ethical review of research projects should assure that the couple "donating" the embryos holds a decisive position; a position which should be respected and included in the process of obtaining embryos for research. In addition, while the recent (August 29, 2000) *National Institutes of Health Guidelines for Research Using Human Pluripotent Stem Cells* allow for federal funding of research using ES cells, they also stipulate that the cells be obtained and derived in respect of certain conditions regarding the donation of embryos for research [3]. Thus, while federal funding is not available for the derivation of ES cells from human embryos, ES cell research may be funded by the US government if certain conditions regarding their derivation, and the manner in which the embryos they were derived from were obtained, are fulfilled.

Is a frozen embryo a live (viable) embryo?

One issue regarding supernumerary IVF embryos that touches the regulatory, scientific and ethical spheres is how long these embryos can and should be cryopreserved. There is, of course, no specific expiration date on embryos, although some countries have determined a limit on the period of time that IVF embryos can be stored. In France, for example, there is a five year limit, and interestingly this is based neither in science nor ethics, but rather serves a legislative aim being set to coincide with the five year revision of the Bioethics Law. At the end of the determined period, the idea is that the couples are asked if they wish to use the embryos in fertility treatment, and if not then the embryos are destroyed.

In the case where frozen embryos are thus destined to be destroyed, can these embryos then be donated for research purposes? Again, this depends on the regulations of the country considered. In the UK, as mentioned above, IVF embryos destined to be destroyed can be donated for research, and it is not considered to be unethical or disrespectful to the embryo.

In France, the possibility of using them in research is an issue for the revision of the Bioethics Law. Since a person cannot be the subject of a donation, however, the question was raised whether or not the frozen embryo is considered to be alive or dead, where the living embryo would be granted personhood, and the dead embryo could be used in research. The argument was made that, considering that freezing is a destructive process in itself, with a possible 50 to 60% loss, a frozen embryo is thus potentially dead. Considering, however, that a frozen embryo is also potentially alive, it is quite difficult to develop the concept of a "legally" dead frozen embryo. After all, who is to say if the frozen embryo is more alive than dead? Finally, and of relevance to this entire discussion, it was pointed out that it would be more appropriate to use the terms "viable" or "non-viable" when discussing frozen embryos, because using "alive" or "deceased" supposes that they have the moral status of the person, which in fact is still at the heart of the debate.

Products of abortion

Going one step further with the above argument, if a frozen embryo is potentially non-viable and destined to be destroyed, then may it be considered equivalent to the products of abortion? In other words, what is the difference between a frozen IVF embryo, that is destined to be destroyed, and the products of abortion? Clearly one major difference is the timing of the destructive act; a frozen IVF embryo is still intact, the products of an aborted embryo are not. It is the consideration that the freezing process may have acted as a destructive act, and rendered the IVF embryo non viable, that inserts doubt here. Going back to the example of France, this kind of distinction would have an impact on the use of these embryos in research, because there is little regulation concerning the use of the products of abortion. It would be difficult, however, as explained by Claire Bonnat-Legras, to consider frozen IVF embryos that are not going to be used in fertility treatment as equivalent to the products of abortion because within the French law IVF and abortion are considered in completely different contexts.

The situation is different in Germany, as presented by Gisella Badura-Lotter, where abortion is theoretically illegal, but tolerated under certain conditions. While there seem to be differences and contradictions concerning the worth of human life between the German abortion law and the Embryo Protection Act, which forbids embryo research, there is in theory no real contradiction. Under the principles of German law the embryo or foetus *in vivo* has the same rights as the embryo *in vitro*.

From both the ethical and regulatory perspectives, an important difference with frozen IVF embryos is that they have traditionally been treated as if they were viable, whereas aborted foetal material is considered non viable. It may seem inconsistent that foetal material may be legally rendered non-viable *via* abortion, and then used for research, without raising the same ethical issues as frozen IVF embryos, which are destined to be destroyed and whose viability is questionable. In other words, from this perspective, the question becomes "should rendering a supernumerary IVF embryo non viable through research be treated differently than rendering a foetus non-viable through abortion?" While this question will not be discussed in depth here, it is at the core of ethical issues facing regulators today.

It is, however, interesting to note that in many cases where a rights based ethic was formerly applied, resulting on a ban on the use of embryos in research based on the principle of non-objectification of the embryo, a shift has occurred and a utilitarian ethic is being considered. The reason for this shift is the staggering therapeutic potential of stem cell technology, considered to promise a medical benefit so large that former rights based arguments on why embryos should not be used in research are being reconsidered. This raises the problem of ethical consistency, both in the case where a rights based ban on embryo research is lifted for utilitarian reasons and in the case where the ban will rest in place whereas the technological benefits (developed elsewhere) will be accepted.

War theory

Looking further into the theoretical basis for ethical arguments, the war metaphor, as we think of the war on disease, was considered as applied to the embryo in research. The question thus raised by one participant is: if a military defence point of view is taken, might we consider embryos as conscripted, for the purposes of survival of individuals that might otherwise die, in the same way that we consider conscripts to war? After all, out of respect for other humans and in order to protect human rights, we accept sending soldiers to war knowing that some of those soldiers will die. Indeed, war theory has been applied to justify the sacrifice of embryos in research in the same way in which we justify the sacrifice of lives by engaging in war. The problem, as explained by Andrew Siegel[1], is that if one considers the viewpoint that the embryo has the moral status of a person, and that the embryo would be an innocent person, war theory doesn't justify killing innocent people. While it is an acceptable side effect of wartime activities that innocent people are killed, it is unacceptable to directly kill and harm innocent people.

With regard to considering embryos as conscripts, war theory does not hold up due to differences in the two scenarios. For example, conscripts are not sent to war with the intention that they will be killed, whereas this would be the case for embryos in research. Also, conscripts have the option of consciously objecting, which the embryo, of course, does not have. While we can justify sending soldiers to war in order to protect human rights (where a violation of human rights has occurred), we cannot use

---

1. In discussion.

human rights to justify sacrificing embryos in research, even though doing so may eventually save lives, because no human right has been violated here.

Regulatory decisions

At the time of this conference, many questions regarding how to regulate research based on stem cells remained open for discussion, with decisions to be made within the months that followed. In the UK, the Chief Medical Officer issued the report on *Stem Cell Research: Medical Progress with Responsibility*, affirming that IVF embryos could be used in research. In the United States, the NIH published their guidelines for *Research Using Human Pluripotent Stem Cells*, upholding the ban on federal funding for embryo research, but extending funding to research on pluripotent ES cells, derived and obtained under certain conditions. In France the 1994 Bioethics law has come up for a mandatory 5 year review. Questions raised by French researchers at regarding the law included: "Today in France, do we have the right to cultivate human ES cells procured from a company?", "Can we receive them for free from a company, or from colleagues?", "Can we be invited abroad to establish the cell lines and then bring them back to France?", and "If not, what is the punishment we will face?" Again, the issue of ethical consistency was raised with the question "If it is illegal for us to procure the cell lines from abroad, will it also be illegal for French people to benefit from the therapies derived from the study of these cells?" Indeed, providing a forum for such questions that were unforeseeable in 1994 was one motivation for including a revision of the Law after 5 years. As remarked by Senator Huriet, despite an interest in keeping up with the development of science, the legislator cannot consider how to best regulate these methods until they actually exist. As discussed here, even when the methods have been developed, science may not hold all of the answers. Regulation is not straightforward and requires a multidiciplinary approach, which can be fostered by gathering people together in fora, such as this one and others.

References

1. Ford N. Are all cells derived from an embryo themselves embryos? In : Dodet B, Vicari M, eds. *Pluripotent Stem Cells: Therapeutic Perspectives and Ethical Issues*. Paris : John Libbey Eurotext, 2001 : 77-83.
2. Mc Lean SAM. Ethical, legal dans regulatory issues in the use of human embryonic stem cells in the United Kingdom. In : Dodet B, Vicari M, eds. *Pluripotent Stem Cells: Therapeutic Perspectives and Ethical Issues*. Paris : John Libbey Eurotext, 2001 : 59-67.
3. Siegel AW. The moral status of the embryo and the politics of human stem cell research. In : Dodet B, Vicari M, eds. *Pluripotent Stem Cells: Therapeutic Perspectives and Ethical Issues*. Paris : John Libbey Eurotext, 2001 : 69-75.

List of contributors

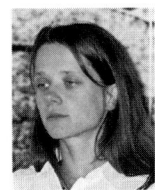

Gisela Badura-Lotter
Lehrstuhl für Etnik in den
Biowissenschaften, Sigwartstr. 20
D-72076 Tübingen,
RFA.
Tel. : 49 70 71 297 75 73.
Fax : 49 70 71 92 28 73.
Email : *gisela.lotter@uni-tuebingen.de*

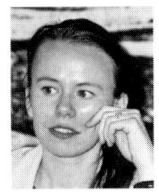

Claire Bonnat-Legras
Conseil d'État,
1, place du Palais-Royal,
75001 Paris,
France.
Tel. : 01 40 20 86 36.
Fax : 01 40 20 80 39.
Portable : 06 80 38 57 51.

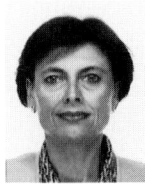

Betty Dodet
Directeur Scientifique,
Fondation Mérieux,
17, rue Bourgelat, BP 2021,
69227 Lyon Cedex 02,
France.
Tel. : 33 (0)4 72 40 79 72.
Fax : 33 (0)4 72 40 79 50.
Email : *bdodet@fond-merieux.org*

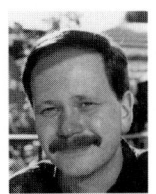

Paul Fairchild
Sir William Dunn School of Pathology,
South Park Road,
Oxford OX 13RE,
Grande-Bretagne,
Tel. : 44 1 865 275 606.
Fax : 44 1 865 275 501
Email : *Paul.Fairchild@path.ox.ac.uk*

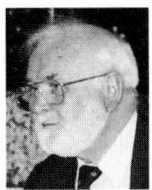

Norman Ford
Caroline Chisholm Centre for Health Ethics,
7th Floor, 166 Gipps Street,
East Melbourne, Vic 3002,
Australia.
Tel. : 61 3 9270 26 81.
Fax : 61 3 9270 26 82.
Email : *nford@mercy.com.au*

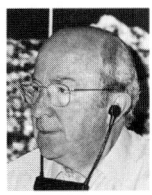

Claude Huriet
Sénat,
Palais du Luxembourg,
Casier Poste,
15, rue de Vaugirard,
75291 Paris Cedex 6,
France.
Tel. : 33 (0)1 42 34 28 82
Email : *churiet@senat.fr*

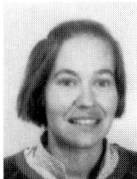

Odile Kellerman
Unité de génétique somatique
(URA, CNRS, 1960),
Institut Pasteur,
25, rue du Dr-Roux,
75724 Paris Cedex 15,
France.
Tel. : 33 (0)1 45 68 85 68.
Fax : 33 (0)1 40 61 31 94
Email : *okellerm@pasteur.fr*

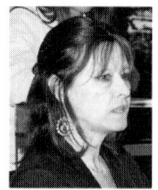

Sheila McLean
Institute of Law and Ethics in Medicine,
University of Glasgow,
University Avenue,
Glasgow G 12 8 QQ,
Scotland. United Kingdom.
Tel. : 44 141 330 36 88.
Fax : 44 141 330 46 98.
Email : *S.A.MMclean@law.gla.ac.uk*

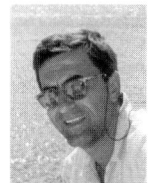

Fulvio Mavilio
Gene Therapy Program,
Istituto Scientifico II. San. Rafaele,
Via Olgettina, 58,
20132 Milano,
Italie.
Tel. : 39 02 264 34701
Fax : 39 02 264 34668.
Email : *mavilio.fulvio@mail.hsr.it*

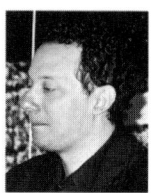

Andrew Siegel
The Bioethics Institute,
Johns Hopkins University,
624N Broadway,
Hampton House 511,
Baltimore MD 21205-1996,
USA.
Tel. : 1 410 955 30 18.
Fax : 1 410 614 95 67.
Email : *Ausphil@aol.com*

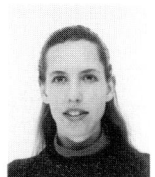

Marissa Vicari
Mapi Research Institute,
27, rue Villette,
69003 Lyon,
France.
Tel. : 33 (0)4 72 13 66 67.
Fax : 33 (0)4 72 13 66 82.
Email : *marissa730@yahoo.com*

Achevé d'imprimer par Corlet, Imprimeur, S.A.
14110 Condé-sur-Noireau (France)
N° d'Imprimeur : 51024 - Dépôt légal : mars 2001
Imprimé en U.E.